W9-BJP-190

Virtual Clinical Excursions

for

Ignatavicius and Workman:
MEDICAL-SURGICAL NURSING:
Critical Thinking for Collaborative Care, 4th Edition

prepared by

Elaine Kennedy, EdD, RN

Virtual Clinical Excursions CD-ROM prepared by

Jay Shiro Tashiro, PhD, RN
Director of Systems Design
Wolfsong Informatics
Sedona, Arizona

Gina Long, RN, DNSc
Assistant Professor, Department of Nursing
College of Health Professions
Northern Arizona University
Flagstaff, Arizona

Ellen Sullins, PhD
Director of Research
Wolfsong Informatics
Sedona, Arizona

Michael Kelly
Director of the Center for Research and
Evaluation of Advanced Technologies
in Education
Northern Arizona University
Flagstaff, Arizona

The development of Virtual Clinical Excursions Volume 1 was partially funded by the
National Science Foundation, under grant DUE 9950613.
Principal investigators were Tashiro, Sullins, Long, and Kelly.

W.B. SAUNDERS COMPANY

An Imprint of Elsevier Science
Philadelphia   London   New York   St. Louis   Sydney   Toronto

W.B. SAUNDERS COMPANY
An Imprint of Elsevier Science

The Curtis Center
Independence Square West
Philadelphia, Pennsylvania 19106-3399

Vice President and Publishing Director, Nursing: Sally Schrefer
Executive Editor: June Thompson
Managing Editor: Michele Trope
Project Manager: Gayle Morris
Designer: Wordbench
Cover Art: Teresa Breckwoldt

NOTICE

Pharmacology is an ever-changing field. Standard safety precautions must be followed, but as new research and clinical experience broaden our knowledge, changes in treatment and drug therapy may become necessary or appropriate. Readers are advised to check the most current product information provided by the manufacturer of each drug to be administered to verify the recommended dose, the method and duration of administration, and contraindications. It is the responsibility of the licensed prescriber, relying on experience and knowledge of the patient, to determine dosages and the best treatment for each individual patient. Neither the publisher nor the editor assumes any liability for any injury and/or damage to persons or property arising from this publication.

Printed in the United States of America

International Standard Book Number: 0-7216-9820-4

02 03 04 05 WB/EB 9 8 7 6 5 4 3 2

Workbook
prepared by

Elaine Kennedy, EdD, RN
Professor, Wor-Wic Community College
Salisbury, Maryland

Textbook

Donna D. Ignatavicius, MS, RNC, Cm
Clinical Nurse Specialist, Calvert Memorial Hospital
Prince Frederick, Maryland
Former Professor, Charles County Community College
La Plata, Maryland

M. Linda Workman, PhD, RN, FAAN
Associate Professor of Nursing
Frances Payne Bolton School of Nursing
Case Western Reserve University
Cleveland, Ohio

Contents

Getting Started

GETTING SET UP

■ MINIMUM SYSTEM REQUIREMENTS

Virtual Clinical Excursions is a hybrid CD, so it runs on both Macintosh and Windows platforms. To use *Virtual Clinical Excursions*, you will need one of the following systems:

- **Windows™**

  Windows 2000, 95, 98, NT 4.0
  IBM compatible computer
  Pentium II processor (or equivalent)
  300 MHz
  96 MB
  800 × 600 screen size
  256 color monitor
  100 MB hard drive space
  12× CD-ROM drive
  Soundblaster 16 soundcard compatibility
  Stereo speakers or headphones

- **Macintosh®**

  MAC OS 9.04
  Apple Power PC G3
  300 MHz
  96 MB
  800 × 600 screen size
  256 color monitor
  100 MB hard drive space
  12× CD-ROM drive
  Stereo speakers or headphones

Ideally, the system you use should have at least 200 MB of free disk space on your hard drive. There are commercially available desktop utility programs that can help clean up your hard drive. No other applications besides the operating system should be running at the time *Virtual Clinical Excursions* is running.

■ INSTALLING VIRTUAL CLINICAL EXCURSIONS

Virtual Clinical Excursions is designed to run from a set of files on your hard drive and a CD in your CD-ROM. Minimal installation is required.

- **Windows™**

  1. Start Microsoft Windows and insert *Virtual Clinical Excursions* **Disk 1 (Installation)** in the CD-ROM drive.
  2. Click the **Start** icon on the taskbar and select the **Run** option.
  3. Type d:\setup.exe (where "d:\" is your CD-ROM drive) and press OK.
  4. Follow the on-screen instructions for installation.
  5. Remove *Virtual Clinical Excursions* **Disk 1 (Installation)** from your CD-ROM drive.
  6. Restart your computer.

- **Macintosh®**

  1. Insert *Virtual Clinical Excursions* **Disk 1 (Installation)** in the CD-ROM drive. The disk icon will appear on your desktop.
  2. Double-click on the disk icon.
  3. Double-click on the icon **Install Virtual Clinical Excursions**.
  4. Follow the on-screen instructions for installation.
  5. Remove *Virtual Clinical Excursions* **Disk 1 (Installation)** from your CD-ROM drive
  6. Restart your computer.

■ **HOW TO USE DISK 2 (PATIENTS' DISK)**

● **Windows™**

When you want to work with the five patients in the virtual hospital, follow these steps:

1. Insert *Virtual Clinical Excursions* **Disk 2 (Patients' Disk)** into your CD-ROM drive.
2. Double-click on the icon **Shortcut to Virtual Clinical Excursions**, which can be found on your desktop. This will load and run the program.

● **Macintosh®**

When you want to work with the five patients in the virtual hospital, follow these steps:

1. Insert *Virtual Clinical Excursions* **Disk 2 (Patients' Disk)** into your CD-ROM drive.
2. Double-click on the icon **Shortcut to Virtual Clinical Excursions**, which can be found on your desktop. This will load and run the program.

■ **QUALITY OF VISUALS, SPEED, AND COMMON PROBLEMS**

Virtual Clinical Excursions uses the Apple QuickTime media layer system. This includes Quick-Time Video and QuickTime VR Video, which allow for high-quality graphics and digital video. The graphics seen in the *Virtual Clinical Excursions* courseware should be of high quality with good color. If the movies and graphics appear blocky or otherwise low-quality, check to see whether your video card is set to "thousands of colors."

Note: Virtual Clinical Excursions is not designed to function at a 256-color depth. (You may need to go to the Control Panel and change the Display settings.) If you don't see any digital video options, please check that QuickTime is installed correctly.

The system should respond quickly and smoothly. In particular, you should not see any jerky motions or unannounced long delays as you move through the virtual hospital settings, interact with patients, or access information resources. If you notice slow, jerky, or delayed software responses, it may mean that your particular system requires additional RAM, your processor does not meet the basic requirements, or your hard drive is full or too fragmented. If the videos appear banded or subject to "breakup," you may need to find an updated video driver for the computer's video card. Please consult the manufacturer of the video card or computer for additional video drivers for your machine.

■ **TECHNICAL SUPPORT**

Technical support for this product is available at no charge by calling the Technical Support Hotline between 9 a.m. and 5 p.m. (Central Time), Monday through Friday. Inside the United States, call 1-800-692-9010. Outside the United States, call 314-872-8370.

A QUICK TOUR

Welcome to *Virtual Clinical Excursions*, a virtual hospital setting in which you can work with five complex patient simulations and also learn to access and evaluate the information resources that are essential for high-quality patient care.

The virtual hospital, Red Rock Canyon Medical Center, is a teaching hospital for Canyonlands State University. Within the medical center, you will work on a medical-surgical floor with a realistic architecture as well as access information resources. The floor plan in which the patient scenarios unfold is constructed from a model of a real medical center. The medical-surgical unit has:

- Five patient rooms (Room 302, Room 303, Room 304, Room 309, Room 310)
- A Nurses' Station (Room 312)
- A Supervisor's Office (Room 301)
- Two conference rooms (Room 307, Room 308)
- A nurses' lounge (Room 306)

■ BEFORE YOU START

Make sure you have your textbook nearby when you use the *Virtual Clinical Excursions Patients' Disk*. You will want to consult topic areas in your textbook frequently while working with the CD and using this workbook.

■ SUPERVISOR'S OFFICE (ROOM 301)

Just like a real-world clinical rotation, you have to let someone know when you arrive on the hospital floor—and you have to let someone know when you leave the floor. This process is completed in the Supervisor's Office (Room 301).

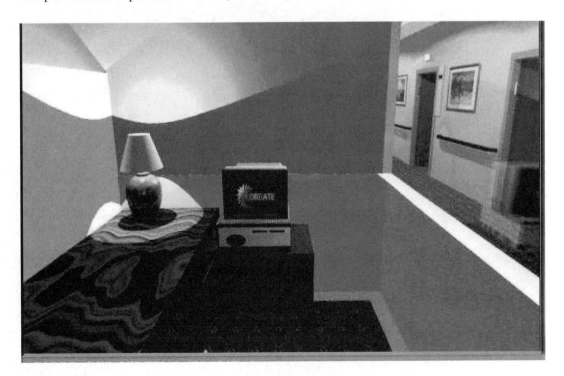

To get a 360° view of where you are "standing":

- Place the cursor in the middle of the screen.
- Hold down the mouse.
- Drag either right or left.

You will see you are in a room with an alcove to your left and a door behind you. To move into the hallway, place the cursor in the door opening and click. Once you are in the hallway, hold down the mouse and make a 360° turn.

In one direction, you will see:

- An exit sign
- An elevator
- A waiting room

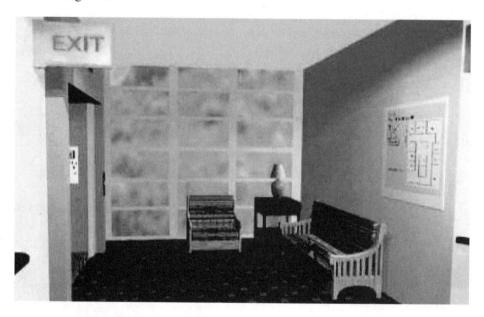

In the other direction, you will see a:

- Patient room
- Mobile computer

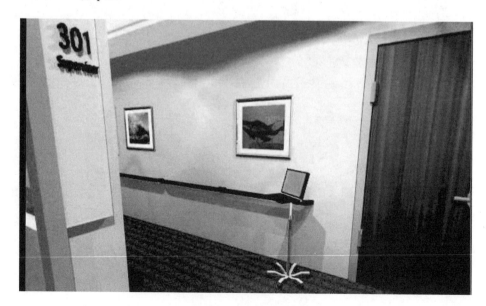

Move the cursor to a new place along the hallway outside the Supervisor's Office and click again. (Always try to place the cursor in the middle of the screen.) You should be moving along the hallway. Remember, at any point you can hold down the mouse and turn 360° in either direction. You can also hold down and move the mouse to the top or bottom of the frame, giving you views looking up or down.

■ READING ROOM

Go back into the Supervisor's Office by clicking on anything inside the room. Explore the Supervisor's Office (Room 301), and you will find another computer. This computer is a link to Canyonlands State University, the simulated university associated with the Red Rock Canyon Medical Center. Double-click on this computer, and a Web browser screen will be launched, which will open the Medical-Nursing Library in Canyonlands State University.

Click on the **Reading Room** icon, and you will see a table of icons that allows you to read short learning modules on a variety of anatomy and physiology topics.

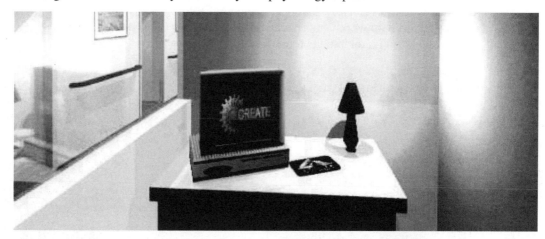

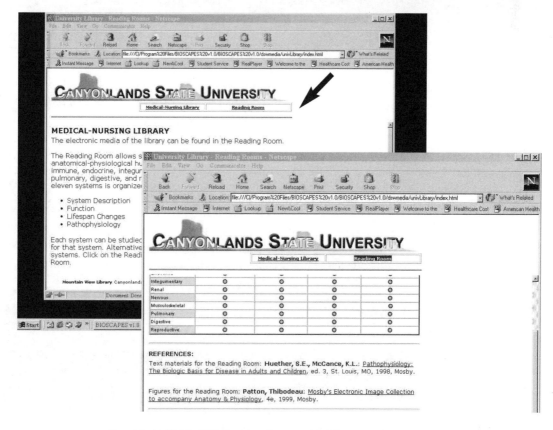

When you are ready to exit the reading room, go to the **File** icon on the browser, look at the drop-down menu, and select **Exit** or **Close**, depending on your Web browser. The browser will close, and once again you will be looking at the computer in the Supervisor's Office.

■ FLOOR MAP AND ANIMATED MAP

Move into the hallway outside the Supervisor's Office and turn right. A floor map can be found on the wall in the waiting area opposite the elevator and exit sign. To get there, click on anything in the waiting area. You should be able to see the map now, but you may not be close enough to open it. Click again on an object in the waiting area; this will move you closer. Turn to the right until you can see the map. Double-click on the map, and you will get a close-up view of the medical-surgical floor's layout. Click on the **Return** icon to exit this close-up view of the floor map.

Compare the floor map on the wall with the animated map in the upper right-hand corner of your screen. The green dot follows your position on the floor to show you where you are. You can move about the floor by double-clicking on the different rooms in this map. If you have already signed in to work with a patient, double-clicking on the patient's room on the animated map will take you right into the room.

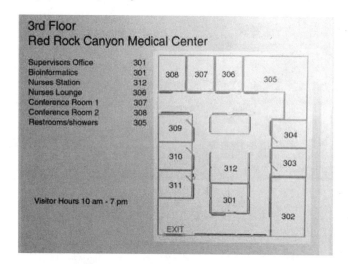
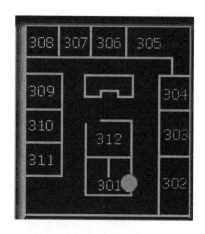

Note: If you have not signed in to work with a patient, double-clicking on a patient's room on the animated map will take you to the hallway right outside the room. If you have not yet selected a patient, you cannot access patient rooms or records.

■ HOW TO SIGN IN

To select a patient, you will need to sign in on the desktop computer in the Supervisor's Office (Room 301). Double-click on the computer screen, and a log-on screen will appear.

- Replace *Student Name* with your name.
- Replace the student ID number with your student ID number.
- Click **Continue** in the lower right side of the screen.

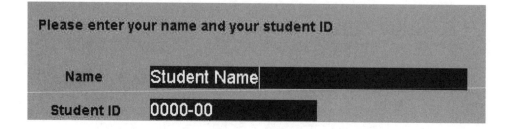

■ HOW TO SELECT A PATIENT

You can choose any one of five patients to work with. For each patient you can select either of two 4-hour shifts on Tuesday or Thursday (0700–1100 or 1100–1500). You can also select a Friday morning period in which you can review all of the data for the patient you selected. You will not, however, be able to visit patients on Friday, only review their records.

■ PATIENT LIST

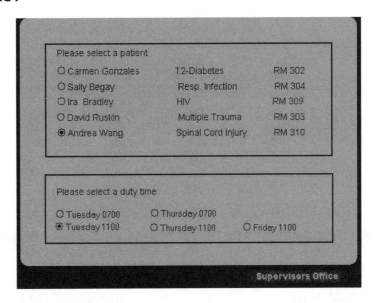

- **Carmen Gonzales (Room 302)**

  Diabetes mellitus, type 2 – An older Hispanic female with an infected leg that has become gangrenous. She has type 2 diabetes mellitus, as well as complications of congestive heart failure and osteomyelitis.

- **David Ruskin (Room 303)**

  Motor vehicle accident – A young adult African-American male admitted with a possible closed head injury and a severely fractured right humerus following a car-bicycle accident. He undergoes an open reduction and internal fixations of the right humerus.

- **Sally Begay (Room 304)**

  Respiratory infection – A Native American woman initially suspected to have a Hantavirus infection. She has a confirmed diagnosis of bacterial lung infection. This patient's complications include chronic obstructive pulmonary disease and inactive tuberculosis.

- **Ira Bradley (Room 309)**

  HIV-AIDS – A Caucasian adult male in late-stage HIV infection admitted for an opportunistic respiratory infection. He has complications of oral fungal infection, malnutrition, and wasting. Patient-family interactions also provide opportunities to explore complex psychosocial problems.

- **Andrea Wang (Room 310)**

  Spinal cord injury – A young Asian female who entered the hospital after a diving accident in which her T6 was crushed, with partial transection of the spinal cord. After a week in ICU, she has been transferred to the Medical-Surgical unit, where she is being closely monitored.

Note: You can select only one patient for one time period. If you are assigned to work with multiple patients, return to the Supervisor's Office to switch from one patient to another.

■ HOW TO FIND A PATIENT'S RECORDS

Nurses' Station (Room 312)

Within the Nurses' Station, you will see:

1. A blue notebook on the counter—this is the Medication Administration Record (MAR).
2. A bookshelf with patient charts.
3. Two desktop computers—the computer to the left of the bulletin board is used to access Red Rock Canyon Medical Center's Intranet; the computer to the right beneath the bookshelf is used to access the Electronic Patient Record (EPR). *(Note: You can also access the EPR from the mobile computer outside the Supervisor's Office, next to Room 302.)*
4. A bulletin board—this contains important information for students.

As you use these resources, you will always be able to return to the Nurses' Station (Room 312) by clicking either a **Nurses' Station** icon or a **3rd Floor** icon located next to the red cross in the lower right-hand corner of the computer screen.

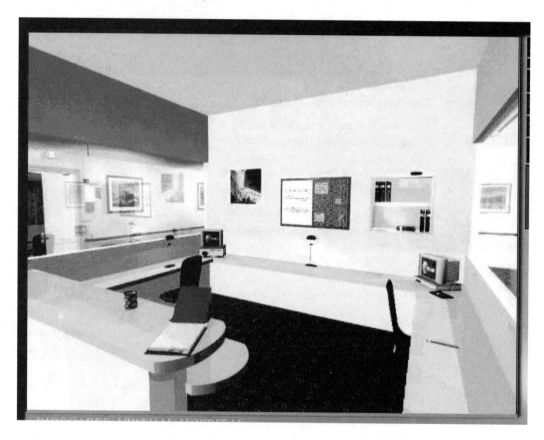

1. Medication Administration Record (MAR)

The blue notebook on the counter in the Nurses' Station (Room 312) is the Medication Administration Record (MAR), listing current 24-hour medications for each patient. Simply click on the MAR, and it opens like a notebook. Tabs allow you to select patients by room number. Each MAR sheet lists the following:

- Medications
- Route and dosage of medications
- Times of administration of medication

The MAR changes each day.

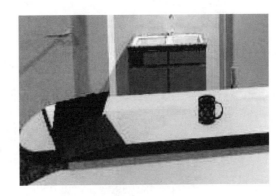

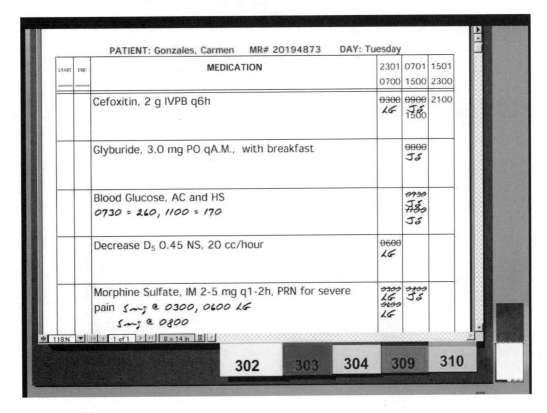

PATIENT: Gonzales, Carmen MR# 20194873 DAY: Tuesday

START	END	MEDICATION	2301 0700	0701 1500	1501 2300
		Cefoxitin, 2 g IVPB q6h	0300 *LG*	0900 *JS* 1500	2100
		Glyburide, 3.0 mg PO qA.M., with breakfast		0800 *JS*	
		Blood Glucose, AC and HS 0730 = 260, 1100 = 170		0730 *JS* 1100 *JS*	
		Decrease D$_5$ 0.45 NS, 20 cc/hour	0600 *LG*		
		Morphine Sulfate, IM 2-5 mg q1-2h, PRN for severe pain *5mg @ 0300, 0600 LG* *5mg @ 0800*	0300 *LG* 0600 *LG*	0700 *JS*	

118% 1 of 1 8 x 14 in

302 303 304 309 310

2. Charts

In the back right-hand corner of the Nurses' Station (Room 312) is a bookshelf with patient charts. To open a chart:

- Double-click on the bookshelf.
- Click once on the chart of your choice.

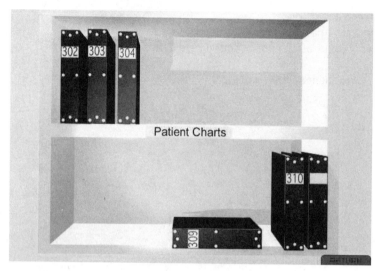

Patient Charts

Tabs at the bottom of each patient's chart allow you to review the following data:

- Physical & History*
- Physicians' Notes
- Physicians' Orders
- Nurses' Notes
- Diagnostics Reports

- Expired MARs
- Health Team Reports
- Surgeons' Notes
- Other Reports

"Flip" forward by selecting a tab or backward by clicking on the small chart icon in the lower right side of your screen. (**Flip Back** appears on this icon once you have moved beyond the first tab.) As in the real world, the data in each patient's chart changes daily.

Note: Physical & History is a seven-page PDF file for Carmen Gonzales, David Ruskin, and Ira Bradley. Physical & History is a five-page PDF file for Andrea Wang and Sally Begay. Remember to scroll down to read all pages.

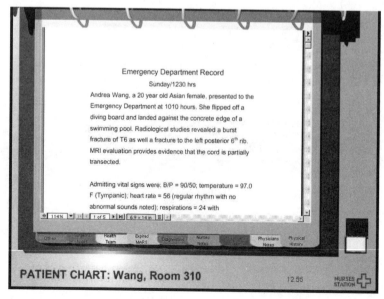

3. Two Computers

◆   **Electronic Patient Record (EPR)**

You can only access an Electronic Patient Record (EPR) once you have signed in and selected the patient in the Supervisor's Office (Room 301). The EPR can be accessed from two computers:

- Desktop computer under the bookshelf in the Nurses' Station (Room 312)
- Mobile computer outside the Supervisor's Office, next to Room 302

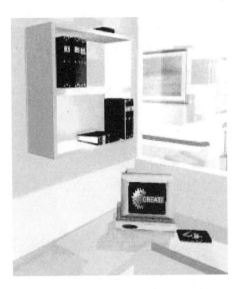
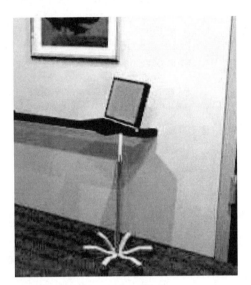

To access a patient's EPR:

- Double-click on the computer screen.
- Type in the password—it will always be **rn2b**.
- Click on **Access Records**.
- Click on the patient's name, then on **Access EPR** (or simply double-click on the patient's name).

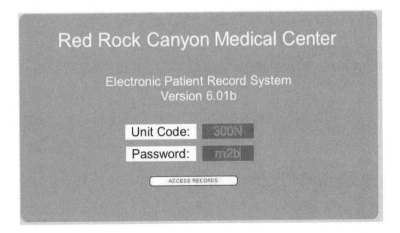

Note: Do **not** *press the Return/Enter key. If you make a mistake, simply delete the password, reenter it, and click* ***Access Records****. You will then enter the records system, where you find a list of patients.*

The EPR form represents a composite of commercial versions being used in hospitals and clinics. You can access the EPR:

- For a patient
- To review existing data
- To enter data you collect while working with a patient

The EPR is updated daily, so no matter what day or part of a shift you are working, there will be a current EPR with the patient's data from the past days of the current hospital stay. This type of simulated EPR allows you to examine how data for different attributes have changed over time, as well as to examine data for all of a patient's attributes at a particular time. The EPR is fully functional (as it is in a real-life hospital or clinic). You can enter such data as blood pressure, heart rate, and temperature. The EPR will not, however, allow you to enter data for a previous time period.

At the lower left corner of the EPR, there are nine icons that allow you to view different types of patient data:

- Assessment
- Admissions
- Urinanalysis
- Vital Signs
- ADL

- Blood Gases
- I&O
- Chemistry
- Hematology

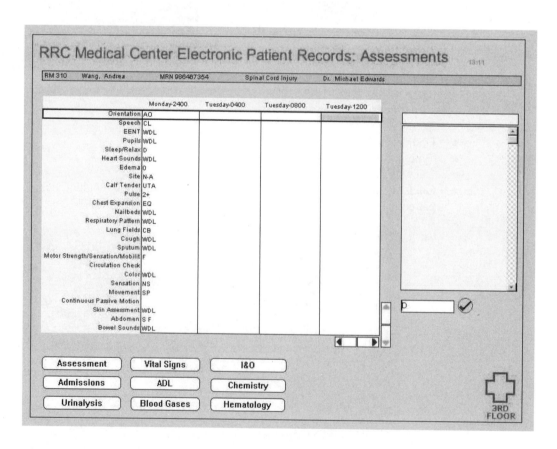

Remember, each hospital or clinic selects its own codes. The codes in the Red Rock Canyon Medical Center may be different from ones you have seen in clinical rotations that have computerized patient records.

You use the codes for the data type, selecting the code to describe your assessment findings and typing that code in the box in the lower right side of the screen, to the left of the checkmark symbol (✓).

Once the data are typed in this box, they are entered into the patient's record by clicking on the checkmark (✓). Make sure you are in the correct cell by looking for the placement of the blue box in the table. That box identifies which cell the database is "looking" at for any given moment.

You can leave the EPR by clicking on the **3rd Floor** icon in the lower right corner. This takes you back into the Nurses' Station (Room 312).

◆ **Intranet**

The computer on the left of the bulletin board in the Nurses' Station (Room 312) is dedicated to Red Rock Canyon Medical Center's **Intranet**. This system contains resources related to working within the hospital. Again, a double click on the screen will activate the computer. A Web browser will come up with four options (Hospital News, Employment, InfoStat, and Home). Navigate within the Intranet just as you would within a Web-based Internet site. Click on **Hospital News** and read some of the articles. The Employment icon opens a screen with descriptions of jobs available in the hospital. The InfoStat icon will connect the hospital Intranet to the Internet. *(Note: This option searches for your Internet connection, activates that connection, and takes you to the publisher's Website for your textbook.)* When in doubt, click on **Home**, which will take you back to the home page for the site.

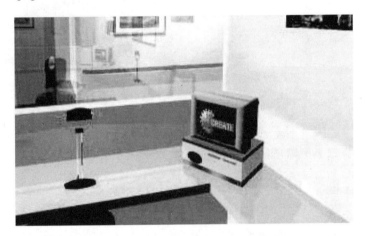

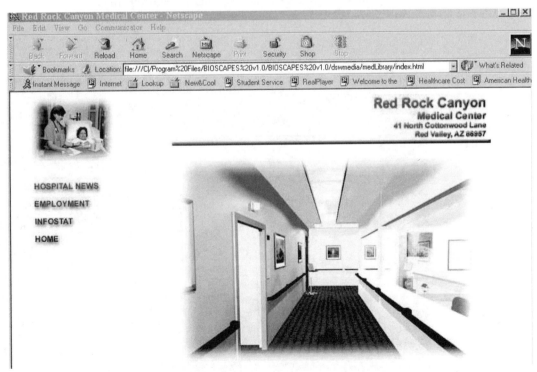

To return to the **Nurses' Station (Room 312)**, exit from the browser. This computer simulates being in a Web environment, so you have to exit from the Intranet by exiting from the browser. Click on **File**, then on **Exit** or **Close** (depending on your browser).

4. Bulletin Board

The bulletin board in the Nurses' Station (Room 312) has important information for students. Click on the board and you can read where reports are being given for patients and where the health team meetings are being held. Lessons in your workbook will direct you to these meetings and reports. Click on **Return** to exit this close-up view of the board.

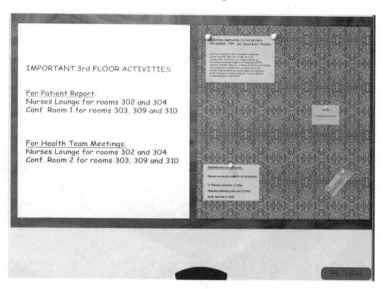

■ VISITING A PATIENT

First, go the Supervisor's Office and sign in to work with Andrea Wang for Tuesday at 0700. Now go to her room. *(Note: The quickest way to get to a patient's room is by double-clicking the room number on the animated map. You can also choose to move through the hallway until you reach the patient's door; then click on the doorknob.)* Once you are inside the room, you will see a still frame of your patient. Below this frame, you will find four icons:

- Vital Signs
- Health History
- Physical
- Medications

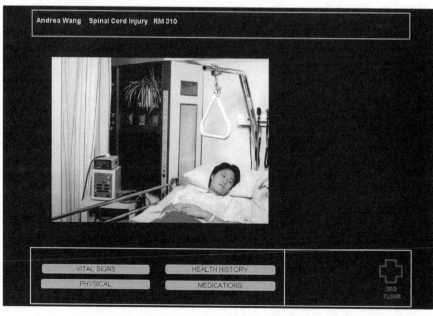

Each of these icons provides the opportunity to assess the patient or the patient's medications. When you click on an icon, you will follow a nurse through the process of collecting assessment data. The nurse will not speak to you but will rely on you to collect the data obtained during patient assessment, to record patient data in the EPR, and sometimes to make decisions after a nurse-patient interaction.

◆ **Vital Signs**

Click on **Vital Signs**; six new icons appear. Each of these new icons allows you to collect data for a particular vital sign. *(Note: You can also see two icons in the right corner.* **Continue Working with Patient** *takes you back to the main menu for this patient. Clicking on* **3rd Floor** *will take you back into the hallway.)* Click on the **Temperature** icon. You will see the nurse take the patient's temperature with a tympanic thermometer. At the end of the measurement, the temperature is shown in the animation of the thermometer to the right of the video screen. These types of interactions allow you to collect data during patient visits.

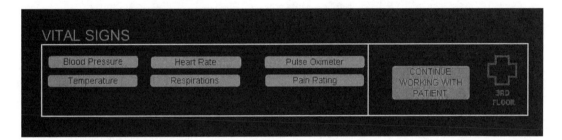

◆ **Physical Examination**

Click **Continue Working with Patient** to return to the main patient menu. Now click the **Physical** icon. Note the different areas of physical examination you can conduct. Try one.

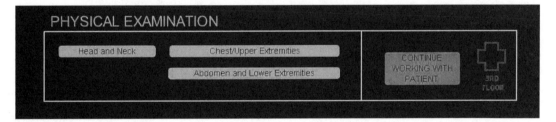

◆ **Health History**

Next, click **Continue Working with Patient** and select the **Health History** icon. In this interactive learning arena, you can ask the patient about her health history. Questions are organized into 12 categories, each of which is accessed by an icon below the video screen. Click on **Culture**, and three new icons appear in the frame to the right of the video. Click on the **Preferred Language** icon, and you will discover the language this patient prefers to use. For each of the 12 question areas, there are three topics you can explore. Thus, there are 36 different question areas related to the health history of each patient.

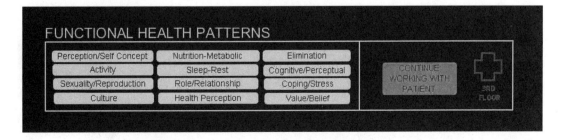

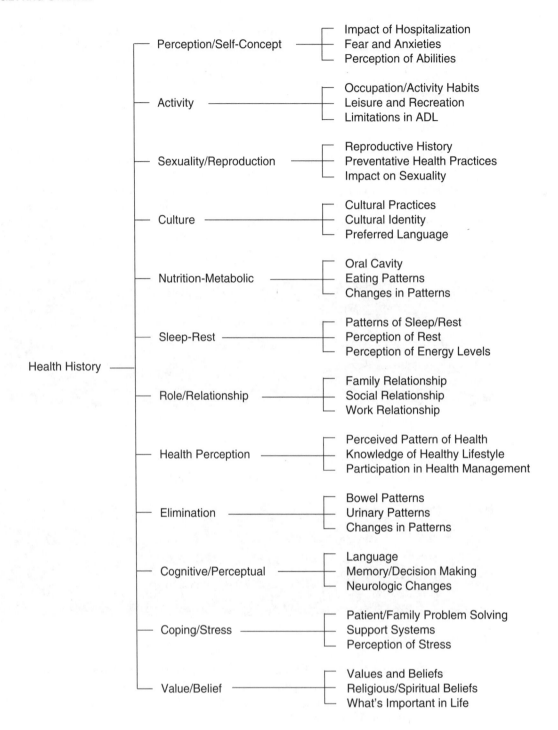

◆   **Medications**

Click **Continue Working with Patient**, and then click the **Medications** icon. Notice that you have three options within this learning environment: Review Medications, Administer, and Hold Medications. Don't click on these now, because you will need to look at this patient's records before you decide whether or not to give medications.

MEDICATIONS

REVIEW MEDICATIONS   ADMINISTER   CONTINUE
                          HOLD MEDICATIONS   WORKING WITH
                                                   PATIENT   3RD
                                                                FLOOR

■ HOW TO QUIT OR CHANGE PATIENTS

How to Quit: If necessary, click either the **3rd Floor** icon or the **Nurses' Station** icon (depending on which screen you are currently using) to return to the medical-surgical floor. Then click on the **Quit** icon in the lower right corner of your screen.

How to Change Patients or Shifts: Go to the Supervisor's Office and double-click on the sign-in computer. Click the **Reset** icon. When the next screen appears, select a new patient or a different shift with the same patient.

A DETAILED TOUR

If you wish to understand the capabilities of the virtual hospital, take a detailed tour by going through the following section.

■ WORKING WITH A PATIENT

Sign in and select Carmen Gonzales as your patient for Tuesday at 0700 hours.

To become more familiar with the *Virtual Clinical Excursions Patients' Disk,* try the following exercises. These activities are designed to introduce you to all of the different components and learning opportunities available within the software. Each exercise will ask you to collect data on a patient.

■ REPORT

In hospitals, when one nurse's shift ends and another begins, the outgoing nurse who attended a patient will give a verbal and sometimes a written summary of that patient's condition to the incoming nurse who will assume care for the patient. This summary is called a *report* and is an important source of data to provide an overview of a patient.

Your first task is to get the report on Carmen Gonzales. Go to the bulletin board in the Nurses' Station. Double-click on the board and check the location where the attending nurse from the previous shift will give you report on this patient. Remember, Carmen Gonzales is in Room 302, so look for that room number on the bulletin board. You will find that the report is being given in the Nurses' Lounge (Room 306). Click **Return** to leave this close-up view of the bulletin board. *(Note: You can also find out where reports are being given by moving your cursor across the animated map.)* Go to Room 306 by double-clicking on the animated map. Once inside the room, click on **Report** and then on **Gonzales**. Listen to report and make a list of this patient's problems and high-priority concerns. When you are finished, click on the **3rd Floor** icon to return to the Nurses' Station.

Problems/Concerns

■ CHARTS

Find the patient charts in the bookshelf to the right of the bulletin board. Double-click on the bookshelf and find Carmen Gonzales' chart (the one labeled **302**). Click on her chart and read the section called Physical & History, including the Emergency Department Record. Determine from this information why Carmen Gonzales has been admitted to the hospital. In the space below, write a brief summary of why this patient was admitted.

■ MEDICATIONS

Open the Medication Administration Record (MAR) by clicking on the blue notebook on the counter of the Nurses' Station. Find the list of medications prescribed for Carmen Gonzales, and write down the medications that need to be given during the time period 0730–0930. For each medication, note dosage, route, and time in the chart below.

Time	Medication	Dosage	Route

Close the MAR and go inside Carmen Gonzales' room (302). Click on the **Medications** icon. You will be responsible for administering the medications ordered during the time period 0730–0930.

To become familiar with the medication options, look at the frame below the video screen. There you will find three opportunities:

- Review Medications
- Administer
- Hold Medications

Click on **Review Medications**. This brings up a frame to the right of the video screen with a list of the medications ordered for the period 0730–0930 hours. Decide whether these medications match what appears within the **Medication Administration Record (MAR)** for this time period. If they do match, you can click the **Administer** icon. If they do not match, you should select **Hold Medications**. When you are finished, click **Continue Working With Patient** to return to the patient care menu.

■ VITAL SIGNS

Vital signs are often considered the traditional signs of life and include body temperature, heart rate, respiratory rate, blood pressure, oxygen saturation of the blood, and the patient's experience of pain.

Inside Carmen Gonzales' room, click on the **Vital Signs** icon. This icon activates a pathway that allows you to measure the patient's vital signs. When you enter this pathway, you will see a short video in which the nurse informs the patient what is about to happen. Six vital signs options appear at the bottom of the screen. Each icon activates a video clip in which the respective vital sign is measured. Relevant vital signs data become available in these videos. For example, click on **Heart Rate**, and a video clip and animation of a radial pulse appear. You can measure the heart rate by counting the animated pulses during a prescribed time.

Try each of the different vital signs options to see what kinds of data are obtained. The vital signs data change over time to reflect the temporal changes you would find in a patient similar to Carmen Gonzales. You will see this most clearly if you "leave" the Tuesday time period you are currently within and "come back" on Thursday. However, you will also find changes throughout any given day (for example, differences between the 0700–1100 and 1100–1500 shifts).

Collect vital signs data for Carmen Gonzales and enter them into the following table. Note the time at which you collected these data.

Vital Signs	Findings/Time
Blood Pressure	
O$_2$ Saturation	
Heart Rate	
Respiratory Rate	
Temperature	
Pain Rating	

After you are done, click on the **3rd Floor** icon in the lower right portion of your screen. This will take you back into the hallway. Move along the hallway (or use the animated map in the upper right corner of your screen) to return to the Nurses' Station. Enter the station, and click on the computer that accesses the Electronic Patient Record (EPR). First you will see the Electronic Patient Record System entry screen. Type in **rn2b** for the password (remember, do *not* press the Return/Enter key). Then click **Access Records**, and you will see a new screen with patients listed. Click on **Carmen Gonzales** and then on **Access EPR**. Now you are in the EPR system. Click on **Vital Signs**, which will open the screen with vital signs data. Use the blue and orange arrows in the lower right-hand corner of the data table to move around within the database. Look at the data collected earlier for each of the vital signs you measured. Use these data to establish a baseline for each of the vital signs.

a. Are any of the data you collected significantly different from the baselines for those vital signs?	Circle One: Yes No
b. If "Yes," which data are different?	

■ PHYSICAL ASSESSMENT

After examining the EPR for vital signs, click the **Assessment** icon and review Carmen Gonzales' data in this area. Once you have reviewed the data and noted any areas of concern to you, close the EPR, enter Carmen Gonzales' room, and click on the **Physical** icon. This will activate the following three options for conducting a physical assessment of the patient:

- Head and Neck
- Chest/Upper Extremities
- Abdomen and Lower Extremities

Click on the **Head and Neck** icon. You will see the nurse conduct an assessment of the head and neck. At the end of the video, a series of icons appear in a frame to the right of the video screen. These icons list the different areas of the head and neck that were examined and the data obtained during the examination. The icons allow you to replay that section of the video in which the particular area was examined.

For example, if you click on **Oculomotor** (the finding is "Oculomotor function intact"), you will see a replay of the assessment of oculomotor function. Each of the icons activates only that portion of the head and neck assessment focused on the particular area described by the icon. The intention is to help you correlate each part of a physical assessment with the data obtained from that assessment—and to give you the opportunity to have the whole assessment of a region conducted beginning to end so that you can learn the process as well as its component parts. Click **Continue Working with Patient** and explore the Chest/Upper Extremities and the Abdomen and Lower Extremities options. For each area, browse through the icons that provide data on a particular area of the assessment. (*Note: The data for certain attributes found during physical assessments change for some patients as you follow them through the virtual week.*)

Focus on the examination of the abdomen and lower extremities by clicking on the option. Pay close attention to the leg wound. In the following table, record the data collected by the nurse during the examination.

Area of Examination	Findings
Abdomen	
Legs	

After you have completed the physical examination of the abdomen and lower extremities, click **Continue Working with Patient** to return to the patient care menu. From there, click on the **3rd Floor** icon and return to the Nurses' Station. Enter the data you collected in Carmen Gonzales' EPR. Compare the data that were already in the record with the data you just collected.

a. Are any of the data you collected significantly different from the baselines for those vital signs?	Circle One: Yes No
b. If "Yes," which data are different?	

■ HEALTH HISTORY

Conduct part of a health history of Carmen Gonzales. Return to her room and click on the **Health History** icon. Twelve health history areas become visible as icons below the video screen. For example, you can see Perception/Self-Concept, Activity, Sexuality/Reproduction, and so on. Note that this patient speaks Spanish and that the nurse has brought in a translator. All of the health history conversations with Carmen Gonzales are completed through translation. Clicking on any of the 12 health history icons reveals three question areas for that category. For example, if you click **Perception/Self-Concept**, a box appears to the right of the video screen with three question areas:

- Impact of Hospitalization
- Fear and Anxieties
- Perception of Abilities

Each of these three areas can be activated by clicking on their respective icons. When an icon is clicked, you will see a video in which your preceptor asks a question in the respective area and the patient answers through the translator.

Since there are 12 health history areas, with three areas of questioning for each, you have access to a total of 36 video clips that provide an opportunity to learn quite a bit about Carmen Gonzales. The questions and responses were chosen for reasons. In fact, conducting an actual health history would not unfold in such discrete and isolated moments; in the real world you would need to follow up some responses with additional questions. Other lessons in this workbook will encourage you to look at each of the health history areas and decide what additional questions need to be asked.

Unlike the vital signs and physical examination findings, the health history data do not change. The developers of *Virtual Clinical Excursions* realized that the number of videos (and the space required for storage) would become too large for the type of educational package we envisioned. We therefore decided to produce only one set of health history data-collecting opportunities. In truth, the health history would probably not change much over a week. Lessons in your workbook may have you collect health history data on the first day of care, or some of the health history queries may be assigned for Tuesday and the others for Thursday.

We recommend that you explore the health history of Carmen Gonzales by choosing some of the 12 categories and asking one or two of the three questions available for each area. When you are done exploring the health history options, leave the patient's room and go to one of the computers that allow you to access the EPR. Browse through the different data fields to see where you would enter data from the health history questions.

Remember: When you are ready to stop working with your *Virtual Clinical Excursions Patients' Disk*, click on the **Quit** icon found in the lower right-hand corner of any of the 3rd floor screens.

■ COLLECTING AND EVALUATING DATA

Each of the patient care activities generates a great deal of assessment data. Remember that after you collect data, you can go to the Nurses' Station or the mobile computer outside Room 302 and enter the data into the EPR. You also can review the data in the EPR, as well as review a patient's chart and MAR. You will get plenty of practice collecting and then evaluating data in the context of the patient's course during previous shifts.

Now, here's an important question for you:

> Did the previous sequence of exercises provide the most efficient way to assess Carmen Gonzales?

For example, you went to the patient's room to get vital signs, then back to the EPR to enter data and compare your finding with extant data. Then, you went back to the patient's room to do a physical examination, and again back to the EPR to enter and review data. If this back-and-forth process of data collection and recording seemed inefficient, remember the following:

- You want to plan all of your nursing activities to maximize efficiency while at the same time optimizing quality of patient care.
- You collect a tremendous amount of data when you work with a patient. Very few people can accurately remember all these data for more than a few minutes. Develop efficient assessment skills, and enter assessment data as soon as possible after collecting them.
- Assessment data are only the starting point for the nursing process.

Make a clear distinction between these first exercises and how you actually provide nursing care. These initial exercises were designed to involve you actively in the use of different software components. This workbook focuses on sensible practices for implementing the nursing process in ways that ensure the highest quality care of patients.

Most importantly, remember that a human being changes through time—and that these changes include both the physical and psychosocial facets of a person as a living organism. Think about this for a moment. Some patients may change physically in a very short time (a patient with emerging myocardial infarction) or more slowly (a patient with chronic illness). Patients' overall physical and psychosocial conditions may improve or deteriorate. They may have effective coping skills and familial support or feel they are alone and full of despair. In fact, each individual is a complex mix of physical and psychosocial elements, and at least some of these elements usually change through time.

Thus it is crucial *not* to think of the nursing process as a simple one-time, five-step procedure:

- Assessment
- Nursing Diagnosis
- Planning
- Implementation
- Evaluation

Rather, it is a creative and systematic approach to delivering nursing care. Furthermore, because all living organisms are constantly changing, we must apply the nursing process over and over. Each time we follow the nursing process for an individual patient, we refine our understanding of that patient's physical and psychosocial conditions based on collection and analyses of many different types of data. *Virtual Clinical Excursions* will help you develop both the creativity and the systematic approach needed to become a nurse who can deliver the highest quality care to all patients.

The following icons are used throughout the workbook to help you quickly identify particular activities and assignments:

 Indicates a reading assignment—tells you which textbook chapter(s) you should read before starting each lesson

 Indicates a writing activity

 Marks the beginning of an interactive CD-ROM activity—signals you to open or return to your *Virtual Clinical Excursions Patients' Disk*

 Indicates additional CD-ROM instructions

 Indicates questions and activities that require you to consult your textbook

LESSON 1 ————————————————

Diabetes Mellitus

————————————————

Reading Assignment: Interventions for Clients with Diabetes Mellitus (Chapter 65)
Patient: Carmen Gonzales, Room 302

You have been assigned to care for Carmen Gonzales, a 56-year-old female admitted to Red Rock Canyon Medical Center with an infected leg that has become gangrenous. She has type 2 diabetes mellitus, as well as complications of congestive heart failure and osteomyelitis.

Pathophysiology

 Before you begin working with the patient, review the pathophysiology of diabetes mellitus in your textbook.

1. Briefly explain the difference between type 1 and type 2 diabetes mellitus.

2. Describe the profile of a patient who has type 1 diabetes mellitus. (See Chart 65-4 in your textbook.)

3. Describe the profile of a patient who has type 2 diabetes mellitus. (Refer to Chart 65-4 in your textbook for help.)

4. Identify the acute complications of diabetes mellitus.

5. Why are the recognition and treatment of these acute changes in blood sugar levels so important?

6. Identify the chronic complications of diabetes mellitus.

Etiology

7. Draw or diagram the sequence of events that typically leads to the onset of type 1 diabetes.

8. What other events could lead to type 1 diabetes?

9. Describe the sequence of events leading to the onset of type 2 diabetes mellitus.

Incidence/Prevalence

 Now apply what you have learned to the case of Carmen Gonzales. On the desktop computer in the Supervisor's Office, sign in to work with this patient for the Tuesday 0700 shift. Then go to the Nurses' Lounge (Room 306) to hear the change-of-shift report. Next, open Carmen Gonzales' chart on the bookshelf in the Nurses' Station and review her Physical & History, including the Emergency Department Record. (Remember to scroll down to read all pages.) When you are finished, access her Electronic Patient Record (EPR) on the computer under the bookshelf. Read her Admissions Profile and review the laboratory data recorded for Sunday at 2000 and 2400.

10. Listed in the right column below are the risk factors for type 2 diabetes mellitus identified in your textbook. Based on your review of Carmen Gonzales' data, use the left column below to indicate whether or not she has each of these risk factors. Identify the specific data you found to support each of your answers.

Carmen Gonzales	Risk Factors
	Family history of diabetes
	Obesity
	Origin
	Age older than 45 years plus any of the preceding factors
	Hypertension
	Previously identified impaired glucose tolerance
	High-density lipoprotein cholesterol level <35 mg/dL (0.90 mmol/L) and triglyceride levels >250 mg/dL (2.82 mmol/L)
	History of gestational diabetes or delivery of babies weighing more than 9 pounds

11. Carmen Gonzales' physical examination in the Emergency Department revealed a blood glucose of 270 mg/dL. The Emergency Department Record also identified various symptoms of which she complained. Which of these symptoms could have been caused by her elevated blood sugar at that time? (See Table 65-4 in your textbook.)

Assessment

12. How do the assessment findings in Carmen Gonzales' Admissions Profile, Physical & History, and EPR laboratory data summaries compare with the expected findings identified in your text? Use Chart 65-17 to complete the flowchart below.

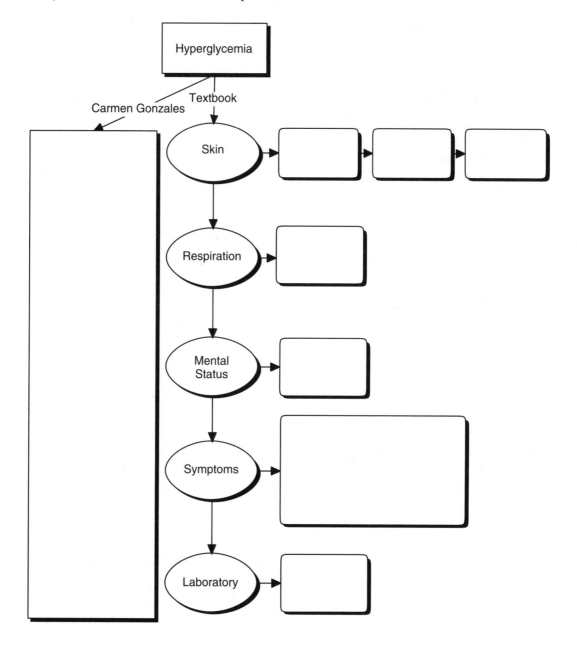

13. Go to Carmen Gonzales' room, take her vital signs, and complete a physical examination of her head, neck, chest, and upper extremities. Record your findings below and in the EPR. While in the EPR, find her blood glucose for Tues 0800 and record under vital signs below.

Tuesday 0800 Findings

Vital Signs

Temperature

Heart rate

Respiratory rate

* Pulse oximetry

Blood pressure

Accucheck

Pain rating, location, characteristics

Head and Neck

Pupils

Oral cavity

Lymph glands

Jugular vein distention

Chest and Upper Extremities

Chest symmetry

Heart sounds

Anterior chest

Posterior chest

Radial pulse

Capillary refill

Hand strength

* A pulse oximeter is a probe used to perform a noninvasive measurement of oxygen saturation. Pulse oximetry (identified in the EPR as SpO_2) is a reliable estimate of arterial oxygen saturation (SaO_2).

Analysis

 Return to Carmen Gonzales' chart and review the physicians' orders for Sunday.

14. Identify the medications that the physician selected specifically for her diabetes mellitus. Consult Chart 65-3 in your textbook if you need help.

 15. What are the classifications for the drugs ordered for Carmen Gonzales' diabetes mellitus?

16. Are the dosages and times ordered for administration of these drugs consistent with recommendations in your textbook or a drug reference book? Explain.

17. When might Carmen Gonzales experience a hypoglycemic reaction following her early morning dose of glyburide and 2U of regular insulin? You will need to consult a drug reference book to answer this question.

18. In the left column below, identify other subclasses of oral hypoglycemic or antidiabetic agents. Give examples for each subclass. In the right column, explain how each of these subclasses accomplishes its hypoglycemic effect.

Oral Antidiabetic Subclass   **Method of Action**

Planning/Implementation

19. Based on the data in the Emergency Department Record, what nursing diagnoses would the admitting nurse have identified for Carmen Gonzales on Sunday evening? Provide a rationale for your answer.

20. On a separate sheet of paper, create a concept map for Carmen Gonzales. For suggestions, refer to the concept map for diabetes mellitus type 2 in your textbook. Be sure to identify the patient's clinical manifestations before you start. Use different colored pens or pencils to develop your concept map. Remember: A concept map is a working tool that grows as information is added. Neatness and artistic ability are not the primary objectives when developing a concept map.

21. The textbook lists six common nursing diagnoses and three common collaborative problems that should be considered when planning care for a patient with diabetes mellitus. Which of these nursing diagnoses and collaborative problems are consistent with your assessment of Carmen Gonzales this morning?

22. What other nursing diagnoses related to diabetes mellitus are suggested by your analysis of Carmen Gonzales' data?

23. Below, prioritize the nursing diagnoses or collaborative problems that you identified in questions 21 and 22 by numbering them from highest to lowest priority. Briefly explain your reason for the order in which you placed them.

24. In the left column below and on the next page, list the first five priority nursing diagnoses or collaborative problems you identified in question 23. (Use both pages and leave plenty of space between entries.) For each entry, select one or two expected outcomes for Carmen Gonzales. Refer to Evaluation: Outcomes in your textbook or a nursing outcomes classification (NOC) manual for help. Then provide appropriate nursing interventions for the outcomes you identified. Finally, offer rationales to explain how these interventions will help to achieve the expected outcomes.

Nursing Diagnosis/ Collaborative Problem	Expected Outcome(s)	Nursing Interventions	Rationale

Evaluation

 Your next task is to evaluate Carmen Gonzales' progress since her admission. First, access her EPR and review her vital signs and assessment data on Sunday at 2400.

25. Below, record and compare the physical examination findings you obtained in Carmen Gonzales' room earlier and the data recorded in her EPR on Sunday at 2000. For any data that were not recorded in the EPR, mark with **NM** (not mentioned).

	Sunday 2400	Tuesday 0800
Temperature		
Heart rate		
Blood pressure		
Respiratory rate		
Lung sounds		
Pain rating, location, characteristics		

 Close the EPR and open Carmen Gonzales' chart. Click on **Expired MARs** and review the notes for Sunday.

26. Below, compare Carmen Gonzales' blood glucose readings and the amount of insulin she was given on Sunday at 2130 (from the expired MARs) with those recorded in the EPR on Tuesday at 0800.

	Sunday 2000	Tuesday 0800
Blood glucose		
Insulin		

 Now return to the EPR and review Carmen Gonzales' I&O data.

27. Using the information documented in the ADL and I&O summaries in the EPR, compare Carmen Gonzales' I&O data for Monday at 0800 and Tuesday at 0800.

	Monday 0800	Tuesday 0800
Appetite		
Oral fluids		
Intravenous fluids		

28. Based on your comparisons in questions 25, 26, and 27, how successful have interventions to combat Carmen Gonzales' diabetes mellitus been to this point? What specific data support your analysis?

29. Below, draw a diagram or concept map to illustrate the associations among Carmen Gonzales' diabetes mellitus and her other medical diagnoses.

30. Based on the associations you found in your diagram or concept map, how important is controlling Carmen Gonzales' diabetes mellitus? Explain.

2

Peripheral Arterial Disease

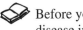 **Reading Assignment:** Interventions for Clients with Vascular Disease (Chapter 36)
Patient: Carmen Gonzales, Room 302

Once again, you have been assigned to care for Carmen Gonzales, a 56-year-old woman who was admitted with an infected leg that has become gangrenous. She has type 2 diabetes mellitus, as well as complications of congestive heart failure and osteomyelitis.

Pathophysiology

Before you begin working with the patient, review the pathophysiology of peripheral arterial disease in Chapter 36 of your textbook.

1. Briefly explain the difference between peripheral arterial and peripheral venous disease.

2. Describe the profile of a patient who has peripheral arterial disease (PAD). (See Chart 36-7 in your textbook.)

3. How does the long-term management of peripheral arterial ulcers differ from that of peripheral venous ulcers?

4. Identify the major complications of peripheral vascular disease.

Etiology

5. Describe the sequence of events that typically leads to the onset of peripheral arterial vascular disease.

6. What other events could lead to peripheral vascular arterial disease?

Incidence/Prevalence

 Please go to the Supervisor's Office and sign in to work with Carmen Gonzales for the Tuesday 1100 shift. Then go to the Nurses' Lounge (Room 306) and listen to the change-of-shift report on this patient. Next, open her chart in the Nurses' Station and read the Physical & History.

7. Based on what you have learned from the change-of-shift report and the Physical & History, what risk factors does Carmen Gonzales have for peripheral vascular disease?

Assessment

8. Complete the chart below to illustrate how Carmen Gonzales' Physical & History assessment findings compare with the expected findings for peripheral vascular disease identified in the text. See Chart 36-7 in the textbook for help.

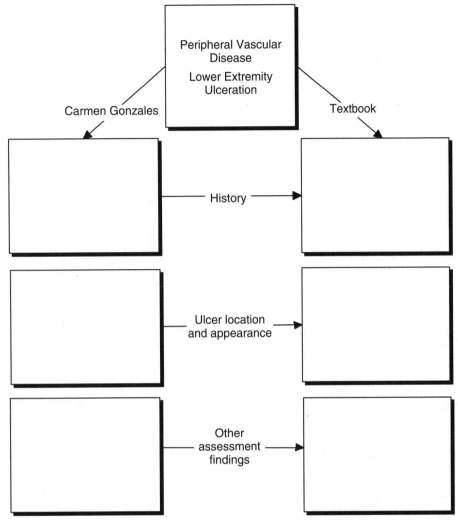

→ Go to Carmen Gonzales' room and complete a physical examination of her abdomen and lower extremities.

9. Use the space below to record your findings from Carmen Gonzales' physical examination. Record your results in her EPR as well.

Abdomen and Lower Extremities	Tuesday 0800 Findings
Bowel sounds	
Palpation	
Edema	
Dorsalis-pedis pulse	
Posterior-tibial pulse	
Skin check	

10. What other assessment data would be useful in evaluating Carmen Gonzales' peripheral vascular disease?

11. Carmen Gonzales has had an open wound on her leg for several days. Why is it important for the nurse to ask how she has been caring for the wound at home?

Analysis

→ Conduct a health history interview in Carmen Gonzales' room.

12. Carmen Gonzales was admitted to the Emergency Department at 1730 on Sunday. Based on her health history interview, what are some possible causes for her symptoms before admission?

→ Return to Carmen Gonzales' chart in the Nurses' Station. Click on **Physicians' Orders** and locate the admission orders for Sunday.

13. Identify the medications that the physician ordered specifically to treat her infection.

14. Are the dosages and times ordered for administration of these drugs consistent with recommendations in your textbook or a drug reference book? Explain.

15. Explain the rationale for giving Carmen Gonzales insulin even though she has type 2 diabetes mellitus and uses an oral hypoglycemic agent at home.

16. What other classes of medications might Carmen Gonzales' physician order for her peripheral arterial disease? Give an example of each class of medication.

Planning/Implementation

17. Given Carmen Gonzales' Emergency Department Record, what nursing diagnoses would the admitting nurse have identified for her on Sunday evening with regard to her peripheral vascular disease?

18. In addition to the nursing diagnoses you just identified, what collaborative problem is suggested by your analysis of Carmen Gonzales' data?

19. Identify the nursing diagnoses/collaborative problems based on your physical exam and health history interview of Carmen Gonzales earlier. (See questions 9 and 12.)

20. Now prioritize the nursing diagnoses or collaborative problems you identified in question 19 by numbering them from highest priority to lowest. Explain your reason for the order in which you placed them.

21. In the left column below, list the nursing diagnoses and/or collaborative problems you prioritized in question 20. (Leave plenty of space between entries.) For each nursing diagnosis you identified, select one or two expected outcomes for Carmen Gonzales. Refer to Evaluation: Outcomes in your textbook or a nursing outcomes classification (NOC) manual for help. Next, provide appropriate nursing interventions for the outcomes you listed. Finally, offer rationales to explain how these interventions will help to achieve the expected outcomes.

Nursing Diagnosis/ Collaborative Problem	Expected Outcome(s)	Nursing Interventions	Rationale

Your next task is to evaluate Carmen Gonzales' progress since her admission on Sunday. Start by accessing her EPR and reviewing her vital signs and hematology data on Sunday at 2400.

Evaluation

22. Below, record and compare the vital signs and physical exam data you obtained in Carmen Gonzales' room earlier (see question 13 in Lesson 1) and the findings recorded in the EPR on Sunday at 2400. (Use **NM** for any data that were not recorded.)

	EPR Data Sunday 2400	Data from Room Visit Tuesday 0800
Temperature		
Heart rate		
Blood pressure		
Respiratory rate		
Pain rating, location, characteristics		

23. Using the information documented in the EPR, compare the pulse oximetry and glucose results from Sunday at 2000 and 2400 with the laboratory results and pulse oximetry results you obtained this morning (see question 13 in Lesson 1). Also record and compare Carmen Gonzales' WBC results documented in the EPR for both days.

	Sunday 2400	Tuesday 0800
Pulse oximetry		
Oxygen source		
Glucose		
WBC		

24. Based on your comparisons in questions 22 and 23, how successful have interventions to combat Carmen Gonzales' infection been to this point? What specific data support your analysis?

25. What further interventions might be implemented to help improve Carmen Gonzales' respiratory status?

Cultural Aspects of Care

Reading Assignment: Cultural Aspects of Health (Chapter 6)
Patient: Carmen Gonzales, Room 302

Continue to care for Carmen Gonzales, this time focusing on the cultural factors that affect her health and the care you give her.

Please go to the Supervisor's Office and sign in to work with Carmen Gonzales for the Tuesday 1100 shift. Access the EPR and review her Admissions Profile. Then go to the patient's room and observe the health history interview, focusing particularly on the categories of Culture and Value/Belief.

1. How does Carmen Gonzales identify herself?

2. Using Purnell's factors for assessing cultural persons (see Table 6-2 in your textbook), identify some health beliefs shared by many Hispanic-Americans. You may need to refer to a sociology textbook in addition to your nursing textbook.

3. How does Carmen Gonzales seem to match the cultural assessment of health beliefs of many Hispanic-Americans?

4. What other areas should be explored with Carmen Gonzales for a more complete cultural assessment?

5. What evidence of spirituality did she voice during her health interview?

6. What questions might you ask to determine whether there are any foods or fluid that Carmen Gonzales prefers or considers unacceptable because of her culture?

7. Identify ways in which these questions or particular questioning approaches might be considered inappropriate by the patient or her family?

8. Use your favorite Internet search engine (if you don't have one, try *http://www.yahoo.com*) and do a search using the key words "Mexican-American culture." Try a second search using "Hispanic culture" and a third search using "Latino culture." Be sure to include the quotation marks. Do you get a different set of sites with each search, or do you get the same sites even though you are using different terms?

9. List some foods that are strongly identified with Mexican-American culture. (Even if you are able to answer this on your own, verify your answer by going to one or more of the websites found in your Internet search in question 8. Remember that the weblinks for your textbook will also provide websites on this topic.)

10. How well do Carmen Gonzales' preferred foods fit the requirements of the diabetic diet and the restrictions of the diet recommended for the control of congestive heart failure?

11. Where did you get your information about Mexican-American foods?

12. How accurate and comprehensive do you think your information source is? On what do you base this opinion?

13. What conclusions can you draw from your searches?

14. How can a health care institution such as an acute care hospital help Carmen Gonzales feel more comfortable?

15. Identify resources or services within your community to which you could refer Carmen Gonzales for help with her therapeutic diet requirements. Ideally, these resources should be familiar with her culture and food preferences and be able to provide information in Spanish.

16. If your community does not have readily accessible assistance for Carmen Gonzales, where can you direct her and her family for information in Spanish?

LESSON 4

Congestive Heart Failure

Reading Assignment: Assessment of the Cardiovascular System (Chapter 33)
Interventions for Clients with Cardiac Problems (Chapter 35)
Patient: Carmen Gonzales, Room 302

For this lesson, you will focus on congestive heart failure and its impact on the health of your patient, Carmen Gonzales, a 56-year-old female admitted with an infected leg that has become gangrenous. She has type 2 diabetes mellitus, as well as complications of congestive heart failure and osteomyelitis.

Pathophysiology

Before you begin working with the patient, review the mechanical properties of the heart (Chapter 33 in your textbook) and the pathophysiology and etiology of congestive heart failure (Chapter 35 in your textbook).

1. Briefly describe cardiac output, heart rate, stroke volume, Starling's law, preload, afterload, and myocardial contractility.

2. State the relationship among cardiac output, heart rate, and stroke volume.

3. Using the relationship you identified in question 2, indicate the changes (↑ or ↓) in cardiac output in the following conditions:

   ↑HR x SV= _____ CO   ↓HR x SV= _____ CO

   HR x ↑SV= _____ CO   HR x ↓SV= _____ CO

4. What compensation must occur to keep cardiac output stable if stroke volume decreases? if heart rate decreases?

5. Use the table below to identify some of the factors that may affect cardiac output, heart rate, stroke volume, preload, afterload, and myocardial contractility.

Factors That May Affect

Cardiac output

Heart rate

Stroke volume

Preload

Afterload

Myocardial contractility

 6. Review the pathophysiology of hypertension (Chapter 35 in your textbook). Briefly summarize the association between hypertension and congestive heart failure.

Please go to the Supervisor's Office and sign in to work with Carmen Gonzales for the Thursday 0700 shift. Open her chart in the Nurses' Station and review her Physical & History. (Scroll down to read all pages.) Also review her Admissions Profile in the EPR.

7. What risk factors does Carmen Gonzales have for decreased cardiac output?

8. What initial compensatory mechanisms does the body use to maintain sufficient cardiac output when problems occur? See Figure 35-1 in your textbook.

9. Complete the diagram below to illustrate the differences between right ventricular failure and left ventricular failure.

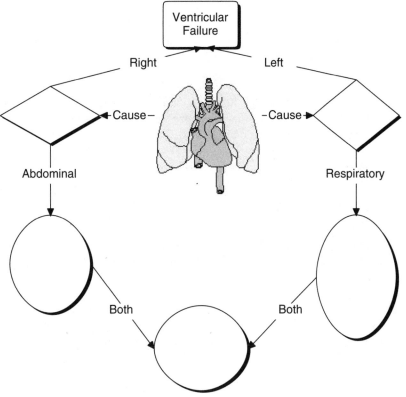

Assessment

10. Complete the chart below to illustrate how Carmen Gonzales' assessment findings on admission to the hospital compare with the expected findings identified in your textbook for a patient with congestive heart failure. Refer to Chart 35-1 and Chart 35-2 in the textbook for help.

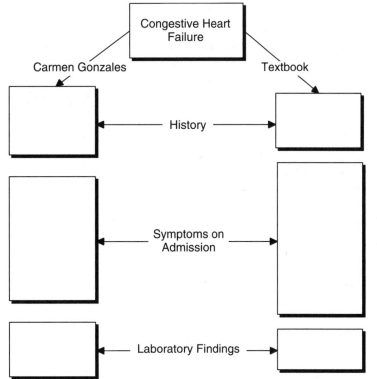

11. Which assessment measure is considered most accurate for assessing fluid retention in patients with dependent edema?

12. If Carmen Gonzales has lost $1\frac{1}{2}$ pounds since she was weighed yesterday, how much water has she lost? (Assume that the entire weight loss was water loss). A handy memory aid is "A pint's a pound the world around."

13. On admission, the nurse noted that Carmen Gonzales was 5 feet 2 inches tall and weighed 170 pounds. What was her weight Tuesday morning? this morning?

14. What would you plan to do in response to your answer to question 13? Why?

→ To complete questions 15 and 16, review Carmen Gonzales' Physical & History and Admissions Profile, as well as the findings from your health history interview and physical examinations from Tuesday 0800 (see Lessons 1 and 2).

Analysis

15. Listed below are several probable nursing diagnoses for Carmen Gonzales. What data from the medical record and from your assessment of the patient support each diagnosis listed?

Nursing Diagnosis	Data to Support Diagnosis
Impaired gas exchange	
Decreased cardiac output	
Activity intolerance	
Ineffective management of therapeutic regimen	
Impaired physical mobility	

Planning

16. In addition to the nursing diagnoses listed in question 15, what other nursing diagnoses and/or collaborative problems do Carmen Gonzales' Admissions Profile, Physical & History, and clinical manifestations suggest related to her congestive heart failure?

17. Below, list all the nursing diagnoses and/or collaborative problems identified in questions 15 and 16. Number them from highest to lowest priority. Explain your reason for the order in which you prioritized them.

18. Your textbook identifies six overall goals for managing the patient with congestive heart failure (listed in the left column below). For each goal, write two expected outcomes. Next, identify appropriate nursing interventions (including medications) for each outcome. Finally, provide rationales to explain how these interventions will help to achieve the expected outcomes.

Goal	Expected Outcome(s)	Nursing Interventions	Rationale
Reduce preload			
Reduce afterload			
Improve contractility			

Maintain ventilation

Maintain nutrition

Psychosocial support

Evaluation

 To gather data necessary to complete the following questions, go to Carmen Gonzales' room, obtain her vital signs, and conduct a complete physical examination. Also search the EPR as needed. (See your answers to question 22 in Lesson 2 to minimize your search.)

19. Compare the physical examination data you just obtained from Carmen Gonzales (Thursday 0800) with the data recorded in the EPR on Sunday at 2400 (Use **NM** for any findings that were not recorded.)

	Sunday 2400	Thursday 0800
Temperature		
Heart rate		
Blood pressure		
Respiratory rate		
Lung fields		

20. Using the information documented in the nurses' notes and in the I&O summary in the EPR, compare Carmen Gonzales' oral intake, output, and the condition of her lower extremities from Sunday at 2400 with the results you obtained from your physical assessment of her abdomen and lower extremities (Thursday 0800).

	Sunday 2400	Thursday 0800
Oral intake		
Output		
Condition of lower extremities		

21. Based on your comparisons in questions 19 and 20, how successful have interventions to improve Carmen Gonzales' congestive heart failure been to this point? What specific data support your analysis?

22. What further information—if it had been documented—would have been useful for purposes of evaluation?

23. What further interventions might be implemented that could help to achieve your desired outcomes?

Older Adults

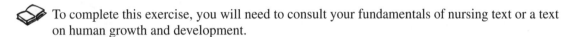

Reading Assignment: Health Care of Older Adults (Chapter 5)
Patient: Carmen Gonzales, Room 302

In this lesson, you will continue to care for Carmen Gonzales, focusing specifically on issues of aging as they affect her health. Remember that she is a 56-year-old female admitted with an infected leg that has become gangrenous. She also has type 2 diabetes mellitus, as well as complications of congestive heart failure and osteomyelitis.

To complete this exercise, you will need to consult your fundamentals of nursing text or a text on human growth and development.

1. What is the primary developmental task of the middle adult as compared with that of the older adult? Give several examples of developmentally appropriate activities for each age group's primary task.

Please go to the Supervisor's Office and sign in to work with Carmen Gonzales for the Thursday 1100 shift. Go to her room and observe the health history interview for the following categories: Perception/Self-Concept and Value/Beliefs. Also, review the assessment data summary in her EPR.

2. Where on the continuum of adult development would you place Carmen Gonzales at this time?

3. Considering the health behaviors that promote wellness in the older adult, which behaviors are appropriate for Carmen Gonzales to demonstrate at this time? (Refer to Chart 5-2 in your textbook for help.)

4. Has Carmen Gonzales experienced any of the common losses of the older adult? If so, identify those losses.

5. Carmen Gonzales' Admissions Profile indicates that she does not have a durable power of attorney for health care or an advance directive on her hospital record. Is it important that her nurse encourage her to consider making her wishes known at this time?

6. What difficulties might the nurse encounter when talking with Carmen Gonzales about advance directives during this hospitalization?

7. What are some developmentally appropriate diversional activities to suggest to Carmen Gonzales? Keep in mind her physical limitations.

8. How might Carmen Gonzales' illnesses affect her growth and development?

9. Compare Carmen Gonzales' risk for falls with the assessment risk factors listed in Chart 5-3 in your textbook. Below, place a **Y** next to each risk factor present in this patient. Place an **N** next to each risk factor that is absent. Record a **?** if you do not have enough information to determine whether a risk factor is present or absent.

Risk Factor	Carmen Gonzales
History of falls	
Advanced age, >80 years	
Multiple illnesses	
Generalized weakness or decreased mobility	
Disorientation or confusion	
Urinary incontinence	
Use of drugs that may cause increased confusion, mobility limitations, or orthostatic hypotension	
Major visual impairments or visual impairments without correction	
Substance abuse	
Location of room away from the Nurses' Station	
Change of shift or mealtime	

10. Is Carmen Gonzales considered at high risk for falls? Why or why not?

11. Does Carmen Gonzales have any risk factors for situational depression? If so, what are they? Provide a rationale for your answer.

12. Why do the normal ranges for laboratory values of many common tests vary from middle adult to older adult? Give two examples of how these normal ranges differ for these age groups. (You may need to consult a clinical laboratory manual.)

13. What implications do age-related changes have for drug administration?

Community-Based Care

 Reading Assignment: Community-Based Care (Chapter 2)
Patient: Carmen Gonzales, Room 302

Continue to care for Carmen Gonzales, this time considering her community-based care needs.

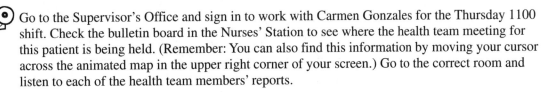 Review Chapter 2 in your textbook.

Go to the Supervisor's Office and sign in to work with Carmen Gonzales for the Thursday 1100 shift. Check the bulletin board in the Nurses' Station to see where the health team meeting for this patient is being held. (Remember: You can also find this information by moving your cursor across the animated map in the upper right corner of your screen.) Go to the correct room and listen to each of the health team members' reports.

1. What type of ambulatory care is Carmen Gonzales likely to use after discharge from the hospital?

2. What are some major responsibilities of the nurse in ambulatory care?

3. Identify the principal concerns related to discharge planning that the nurse case manager reports in the team meeting.

4. Identify the major concern voiced by the clinical nurse specialist related to Carmen Gonzales' discharge plan.

5. Identify the main concerns that the social worker has for Carmen Gonzales' discharge plan.

6. Are the health care needs identified for Carmen Gonzales by the heath team members appropriate for management by a nurse in ambulatory care? Explain.

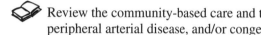 Review the community-based care and teaching necessary for patients with diabetes mellitus, peripheral arterial disease, and/or congestive heart failure as discussed in Chapters 35, 36, and 65 of your textbook.

7. Based on your textbook reading and your answers to questions 3, 4, and 5, complete the following chart addressing Carmen Gonzales' community-based care needs.

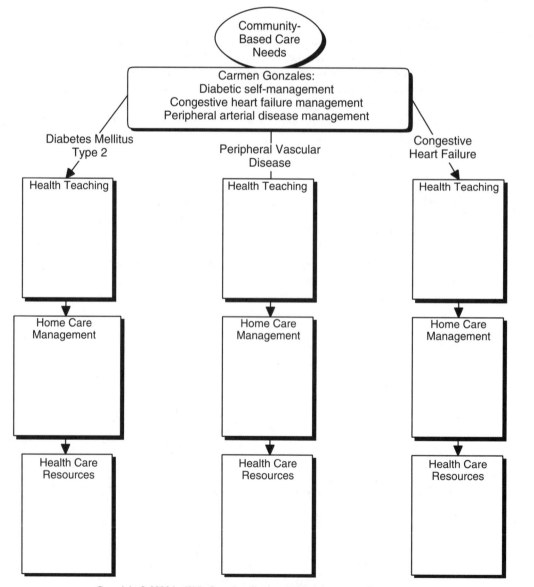

8. What information should be included in a discharge plan for Carmen Gonzales to prevent future infections? (Refer to Chart 65-8 in your textbook.)

9. Based on the items you included in your plan of care for Carmen Gonzales in question 7, what outcome measures would you want to document?

Evaluation of Care

Reading Assignment: Interventions for Clients with Cardiac Problems (Chapter 35)
Interventions for Clients with Malnutrition and Obesity
(Chapter 36)
Patient: Carmen Gonzales, Room 302

Your patient, Carmen Gonzales, will soon be discharged. As her nurse, it will be your responsibility to make sure that she has all the needed information regarding her immediate care after hospitalization. Remember that she is 56 years old and was admitted with an infected leg that has become gangrenous. She also has type 2 diabetes mellitus, as well as complications of congestive heart failure and osteomyelitis.

1. What is the overall goal for the care of older patients with diabetes mellitus?

2. What information needs to be included in a discharge nurse's note for Carmen Gonzales' medical record?

In the Supervisor's Office, sign in to work with Carmen Gonzales for the Thursday 1100 shift. Go to the Nurses' Lounge (Room 306) and listen to the health team meeting.

3. The clinical nurse specialist and the nurse case manager both express concern about Carmen Gonzales' cardiac status in addition to her diabetes mellitus. Identify at least three ways that her history of myocardial infarction and congestive heart failure affect the management of her diabetes.

4. What information about medications should be given to Carmen Gonzales?

5. In your textbook, review the evaluation outcomes for diabetes mellitus, peripheral arterial disease, and congestive heart failure (see Chapters 35, 36, and 65). In the left column below, list the expected outcomes suggested for each disease. (You will fill in other columns in question 6.)

Expected Outcomes	Nurses' Notes	Physicians' Notes	EPR
Diabetes mellitus			
Peripheral arterial disease			
Congestive heart failure			

→ Go to the Nurses' Station and open Carmen Gonzales' chart. Review the nurses' notes and physicians' notes, looking for evidence that indicates whether or not the outcomes suggested by your textbook have been achieved in her case. Then access her EPR and search for the same evidence in her data summaries.

6. Record your findings on the chart in question 5 on the previous page. Next to each outcome, under the corresponding CD source of data, record a **Y** if you found evidence of outcome attainment, record an **N** if you found evidence that the outcome had not been achieved, and record **NM** if the outcome was not mentioned.

7. Based on your chart in question 5, what outcomes need to be evaluated and noted?

8. Now that you have reviewed the data documented in Carmen Gonzales' chart and EPR and listened to the health team members' concerns, what health problem has been overlooked during her hospitalization?

9. How might the nurse discharging Carmen Gonzales remedy this oversight?

LESSON 8

Pneumonia

 Reading Assignment: Assessment of the Respiratory System (Chapter 27)
Intervention for Clients with Infectious Respiratory Problems
(Chapter 31)
Patient: Sally Begay, Room 304

For this lesson, you have been assigned to care for Sally Begay, a 58-year-old female admitted with respiratory distress and fever of unknown origin, rule out Hantavirus.

Pathophysiology

Before you begin, review the pathophysiology of pneumonia in Chapter 31 of your textbook.

1. Briefly summarize the three major pathologic changes that occur in the lung.

2. List the two ways that the textbook classifies pneumonias. What type of pneumonia does Sally Begay most likely have?

Please sign in to work with Sally Begay for the Tuesday 0700 shift. Go to listen to her change-of-shift report in Room 306. After listening to the report, review the Physical & History in her chart in the Nurses' Station. (Scroll down to read all pages.)

3. What discrepancies did you note between the two sources of information on Sally Begay?

4. Do any of these discrepancies make a significant difference in planning nursing care for Sally Begay?

5. How can you verify which data are correct?

Incidence/Prevalence

6. After reading Sally Begay's Physical & History, compare her risk factors for pneumonia with those identified in Table 31-3 in your textbook. Which risk factors does she have?

7. What items should the nurse plan to include in Sally Begay's discharge instructions to decrease her risk factors?

Assessment

8. Complete the chart below to illustrate how Sally Begay's assessment findings in her chart compare with the expected findings identified in the textbook. Consult Table 31-6 for help.

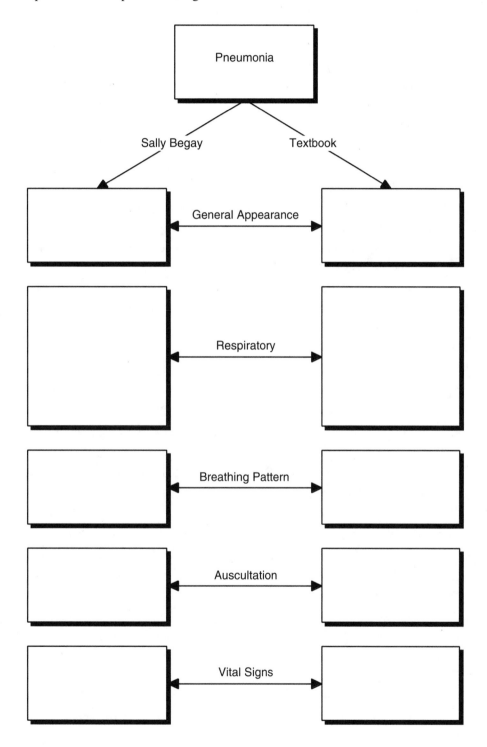

→ Access Sally Begay's EPR and review her vital signs and blood gas reports.

9. Sally Begay was admitted to the Emergency Department on Saturday at 1200. Based on the EPR data, for each of the times listed below, record her arterial blood gas values for oxygen (PaO_2) and pulse oximetry. Also indicate the amount of supplemental oxygen she is using at each time. Use **NM** if no reports are available.

	Sat 1600	Sat 2000	Sun 1600	Mon 1600
Arterial oxygen (PaO_2)				
Pulse oximetry				
Supplemental oxygen				

10. If you were the nurse admitting Sally Begay and you obtained a value for pulse oximetry of 87%, what other data would you want to collect?

11. Is Sally Begay's admitting chest x-ray consistent with the tentative medical diagnosis of pneumonia? Explain.

Go to Sally Begay's room, take her vital signs, and conduct a physical examination of the chest and upper extremities.

12. Below, record the data you obtained during your room visit with Sally Begay. Document these findings in the EPR as well.

Tuesday 0800 Findings

Respiratory rate

Heart rate

Temperature

Blood pressure

Pulse oximetry

Pain rating, location, characteristics

Chest expansion

Respiratory pattern

Lung fields

Cough

Sputum

Oxygen source

13. Are the data you collected related to Sally Begay's respiratory status consistent with a diagnosis of pneumonia as outlined in the textbook?

14. During your visit with Sally Begay, you should have noticed that she had pink nail polish on her fingers. What effect, if any, might the nail polish have had on the accuracy of the pulse oximetry reading?

Analysis

15. What are two common nursing diagnoses for patients with pneumonia?

16. What data from Sally Begay's chart and from your physical examination and vital signs findings support each of the nursing diagnoses listed below?

Nursing Diagnosis	Data from Physical Examination and Vital Signs	Data from Patient's Chart
Impaired gas exchange		
Ineffective airway clearance		

17. A common collaborative problem with pneumonia is CP: Sepsis related to an infectious organism. What risk factors does Sally Begay have that increase her risk for sepsis? (See Table 31-3 in your textbook if you need help.)

18. Chapter 31 in your textbook lists five other nursing diagnoses that should be considered when planning care for a patient with pneumonia. Which of these additional nursing diagnoses are consistent with your assessment of Sally Begay?

In Sally Begay's chart, locate and review the physician's admission orders on Sunday.

19. Identify the medications that the physician ordered specifically to combat pneumonia. (Consult Chart 31-7 in your textbook for help.)

20. What is the classification for the drugs you identified in question 19?

21. Are the dosages and times ordered for administration of these drugs consistent with recommendations in your drug reference book? If not, explain.

22. Which other drug ordered by the physician should aid in improving respiratory function?

23. How does this drug aid respiratory function?

24. What information is missing from the acetaminophen (Tylenol™) order?

Planning/Implementation

 25. Refer to the concept map entitled Bacterial Pneumonia in the Elderly in Chapter 31 of your textbook for suggestions for developing a clinical correlation map. Using this example, develop your own clinical correlation map for Sally Begay on a separate sheet of paper.

26. Identify the risk factors that Sally Begay has for bacterial pneumonia.

27. Which clinical manifestations of bacterial pneumonia does Sally Begay exhibit?

28. In addition to Impaired gas exchange and Ineffective airway clearance, what other nursing diagnoses and/or collaborative problems for Sally Begay are suggested by your analysis?

29. List all of the potential nursing diagnoses and collaborative problems that have been identified or suggested for Sally Begay. (Include Impaired gas exchange, Ineffective airway clearance, and those you listed in question 28.) Number them from highest to lowest priority.

30. In the left column below, list the nursing diagnoses and collaborative problems you identified in question 29. (Leave plenty of space between entries.) For each diagnosis or collaborative problem, select one or two expected outcomes for Sally Begay. Refer to Evaluation: Outcomes in the textbook or an NOC manual for help. Next, provide appropriate nursing interventions for the outcomes you identified. Consult Chart 31-5 in your textbook or a nursing interventions classification (NIC) manual if you need help. Finally, offer rationales to explain how these interventions will help to achieve the expected outcomes.

Nursing Diagnosis/Collaborative Problem	Expected Outcome(s)	Nursing Interventions	Rationale

Return to Sally Begay's EPR and review her vital signs and assessment data for Saturday at 1600.

Evaluation

31. Below, record your findings from the EPR for each of the vital signs and physical examination areas listed. Also record the data you obtained earlier in Sally Begay's room (see your answer to question 12 for this data).

	EPR Data Saturday 1600	Data from Room Visit Tuesday 0800
Temperature		
Heart rate		
Blood pressure		
Respiratory rate		
Pain rating, source, characteristics		
Respiratory pattern		
Lung sounds		
Cough		
Sputum		

32. Using the information documented in the EPR vital signs summary, compare the pulse oximetry and oxygen readings from Saturday at 2000 with the results you obtained in question 12 of this lesson (Tuesday 0800).

	Saturday 2000	Tuesday 0800
Pulse oximetry		
Oxygen source		

➤ Return to Sally Begay's EPR and click on **Hematology**.

33. Below, record Sally Begay's white blood cell count (WBC) on Saturday at 1600 and Tuesday at 0800.

	Saturday 1600	Tuesday 0800
WBC		

34. Based on your comparisons in questions 31, 32, and 33, how successful have interventions to combat Sally Begay's pneumonia been to this point? What specific data support your analysis?

35. What further interventions could be implemented to help achieve your desired outcomes?

LESSON 9

Pain

Reading Assignment: Pain: The Fifth Vital Sign (Chapter 7)
Patient: Sally Begay, Room 304

Continue caring for Sally Begay, this time focusing on the pain she is experiencing. In the Supervisor's Office, sign in to work with her for the Tuesday 1100 shift. Go to her room and obtain a complete set of vital signs. Also review the Physical & History in her chart as needed to answer questions in this lesson.

Review the pathophysiology of pneumonia in Chapter 31 of your textbook.

1. Given the pathophysiology of pneumonia, what is the most likely source of Sally Begay's pain?

2. What specific factors in her health history may influence her perceptions of pain?

3. What type of pain is Sally Begay probably experiencing?

4. What specific data gathered from the patient supports your analysis of the type of pain that she is experiencing?

87

ASSESSMENT

5. According to her Physical & History, how long has Sally Begay been experiencing her pain?

6. When the nurse asks Sally Begay to rate her pain, what assessment tool is the nurse using? See Figure 7-4 in your textbook for help.

7. How should the pain rating scale be described to the patient?

ANALYSIS

8. How easy do you think it is for Sally Begay to describe the pain sensation she is experiencing?

9. How easy do you think it is for her to locate where the pain is occurring?

10. Review the elements of a complete pain history in Chapter 7 of your textbook. How complete is the documentation regarding Sally Begay's pain? Are precipitating factors, aggravating factors, localization of pain, character and quality of pain, and duration of pain clearly stated? Explain. (You will need to review all relevant sources of data on your CD-ROM to make an assessment.)

11. Identify where you found the information necessary to answer question 10.

PLANNING/IMPLEMENTATION

12. What nursing diagnoses or collaborative problems would you select for Sally Begay based on her pain assessment?

 13. What outcome measures will indicate success in managing Sally Begay's pain? Review Evaluation: Outcomes in the textbook or an NOC manual under Comfort Level, Pain Control, Pain: Disruptive Effects, or Pain Level for suggestions.

14. Explain why Sally Begay's physician did not order a cough suppressant to alleviate the pain she is experiencing from her productive cough. Review Chart 31-5 in your textbook for NIC intervention activities for cough enhancement.

15. What interventions other than medications may help alleviate Sally Begay's pain?

16. Explain why your selected interventions should help decrease Sally Begay's pain.

EVALUATION

→ Access Sally Begay's EPR, click on **Vital Signs**, and locate the data related to her pain.

17. Below, record Sally Begay's pain ratings from Saturday at 2000 through Tuesday at 0400. Also record the source and characteristics of her pain for each time.

	Sat 2000	Sun 1200	Mon 1200	Tues 0400
Pain rating				
Pain source				
Pain characteristics				

18. Based on your comparison of Sally Begay's pain in question 17, how successful have interventions to combat her pain been to this point?

19. What specific data support your analysis?

20. What further interventions might be implemented to help achieve the desired outcomes?

Cultural Aspects of Care

/⊙⊙ **Reading Assignment:** Cultural Aspects of Health (Chapter 6)
Patient: Sally Begay, Room 304

This lesson focuses on the cultural aspects of health and how they affect the care you provide for your patient, Sally Begay.

⊙ In the Supervisor's Office, sign in to work with Sally Begay on Tuesday at 1100. Then go to one of the computers that allow you to access the EPR. Open Sally Begay's EPR and read her Admissions Profile. Next, visit the patient in her room and conduct a complete health history interview in the categories of Culture and Value/Belief.

1. How does Sally Begay identify herself?

2. What evidence of spirituality does she voice during her health interview?

3. How do you interpret the patient's statements that she is Diné and tries "to keep the traditional ways"?

4. Sally Begay needs to increase her fluid intake. Suggest several ways to determine her fluid preferences.

5. Speculate how any of your possible approaches to gathering information might be considered inappropriate or unacceptable to Sally Begay or her family.

6. Use your favorite Internet search engine (if you don't have one, try *http://www.yahoo.com*) and do a search using the key words "Navajo culture." Be sure to include the quotation marks. Use the space below to list websites you find.

7. List some common Navajo food preferences. (Even if you are able to answer this on your own, verify your answer by going to one or more of the websites found in your Internet search in question 6. Remember that the weblinks for your textbook will also provide websites on this topic.)

8. Where did you get your information about Navajo food preferences?

9. How accurate do you think your information source is? On what do you base your opinion?

10. What cultural practice does Sally Begay plan to use to help restore her health?

11. How can a health care institution such as an acute care hospital help Sally Begay feel more comfortable?

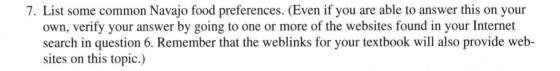 Return to Sally Begay's room, click on **Physical Examination**, then on **Chest/Upper Extremities**, and observe the nurse listening to her heart sounds and breath sounds.

12. What evidence indicates that the nurse is being respectful of Sally Begay?

11

Chronic Bronchitis and Tuberculosis

 Reading Assignment: Interventions for Clients with Noninfectious Lower Respiratory Problems (Chapter 30)
Interventions for Clients with Infectious Respiratory Problems (Chapter 31)

Patient: Sally Begay, Room 304

In this lesson, you will review issues related to chronic bronchitis and tuberculosis and apply what you have learned to the case of Sally Begay.

Pathophysiology

Review the pathophysiology, etiology, and incidence/prevalence of chronic bronchitis and pulmonary tuberculosis in Chapters 30 and 31 of your textbook.

1. Briefly summarize the major pathologic changes that occur in the lung with chronic bronchitis.

2. What are the most common causes for chronic bronchitis?

Sign in to work with Sally Begay on Thursday at 0700. Review the Physical & History in her chart, as well as her Admissions Profile in the EPR.

3. Which, if any, of the causes for chronic bronchitis applies to Sally Begay's condition?

4. What evidence supports the medical diagnosis of emphysema and chronic bronchitis?

5. Explain the relationship between chronic bronchitis and emphysema.

6. Briefly summarize the major pathologic changes that occur in the lung with pulmonary tuberculosis.

→ Browse through various sections of Sally Begay's chart and look for documentation of any of the pathologic changes you identified in question 6.

7. What evidence in the chart supports the medical diagnosis of pulmonary tuberculosis for this patient? Where did you find this data?

Incidence/Prevalence

8. The Admissions Profile and Physical & History for Sally Begay contain incomplete information about one important fact needed to plan care for managing chronic respiratory illnesses. What information should be included?

9. Compare Sally Begay's risk factors for pulmonary tuberculosis with those identified in Chapter 30 of your textbook. Which risk factors does she have?

10. Identify three items that the nurse should plan to include in Sally Begay's discharge instructions to decrease her risk for recurrent pulmonary tuberculosis.

Assessment

→ To complete questions 11 and 12, read the diagnostic reports in Sally Begay's chart. Then access the EPR and review the data recorded on Saturday at 1600 for hematology, chemistry, and blood gases.

11. Complete the chart below to illustrate how Sally Begay's laboratory and radiographic findings on admission compare with the expected findings identified in the textbook for a patient with COPD. In the center boxes, record the normal value ranges for each diagnostic test listed. In the box to the left of each test, record your findings from the EPR. To the right of each test, indicate the expected findings identified in Chapter 30 in your textbook.

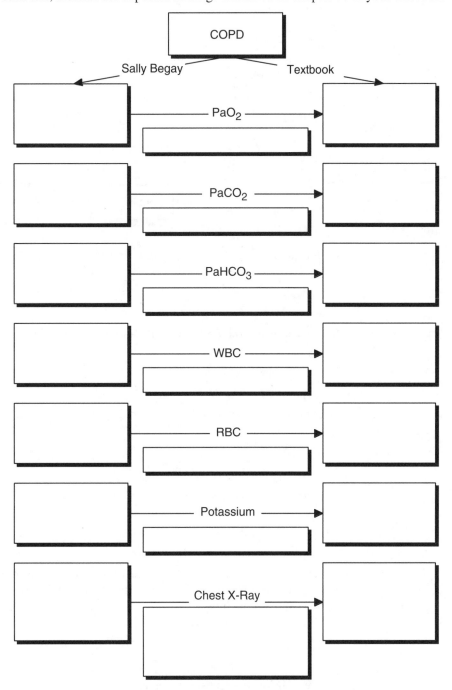

12. Which of the laboratory and radiographic findings on admission are also consistent with the primary diagnosis of pneumonia for Sally Begay?

13. Use the Venn comparison diagram below to answer questions *a–d* concerning the symptoms of pneumonia, COPD, and pulmonary tuberculosis. Refer to discussions on clinical manifestations in your textbook for help.

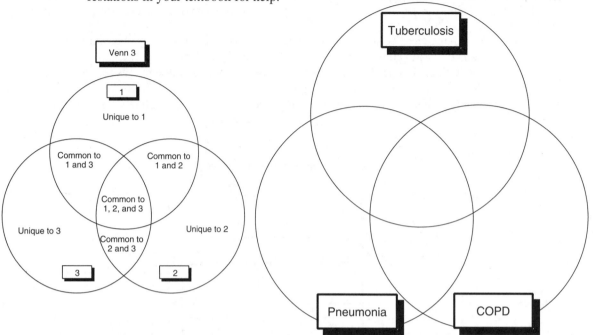

a. Identify the clinical manifestations that all three respiratory illnesses share.

b. Identify the clinical manifestations that are the same for pneumonia and tuberculosis.

c. Identify the clinical manifestations that are shared by pneumonia and COPD.

d. Identify the clinical manifestations that are the same for COPD and tuberculosis.

14. Based on the Venn comparison diagram, which one of the following respiratory symptoms is unique to pulmonary tuberculosis: night sweats, anorexia, weight loss, shortness of breath, cough, or sputum production?

15. What diagnostic test positively identifies tuberculosis?

Analysis

 16. What are two common nursing diagnoses for patients with COPD and pulmonary tuberculosis?

→ Go to Sally Begay's room and conduct a health history interview. Focus particularly on the categories of Sleep-Rest and Activity. Then review her chart and EPR as needed to complete question 17.

17. What data from the chart and/or EPR and from your interview with Sally Begay support each of the nursing diagnoses listed below? Identify where you found your answers.

Nursing Diagnoses	Health History Data	Chart and/or EPR Data
Fatigue		
Activity intolerance		

→ In Sally Begay's chart, locate and review the physician's admission orders for Saturday.

18. Identify the medication that the physician ordered specifically to treat Sally Begay's chronic bronchitis and COPD. Consult Table 30-3 in your textbook if you need help.

19. What is the classification for the drug you identified in question 18?

20. Are the dosages and times ordered for administration of this drug consistent with recommendations in the textbook?

21. For what side effects of albuterol should the nurse be observing Sally Begay?

Planning

22. Which clinical manifestations of chronic bronchitis does Sally Begay have?

23. In addition to Fatigue and Activity intolerance, what other nursing diagnoses do Sally Begay's Admissions Profile, Physical & History, and clinical manifestations suggest?

24. Prioritize the nursing diagnoses you identified in question 23 by numbering them from highest to lowest priority. Provide a rationale for the order in which you placed them.

25. In the left column below, list the three highest priority nursing diagnoses from question 24. (Leave plenty of space between entries.) For each diagnosis, select one or two expected outcomes for Sally Begay. Next, offer appropriate nursing interventions for the outcomes you identified. (Consult Chart 30-7 in your textbook or an NIC manual for interventions.) Finally, provide rationales to explain how these interventions will help to achieve the expected outcomes.

Nursing Diagnosis/ Collaborative Problem	Expected Outcome(s)	Nursing Interventions	Rationale

Evaluation

 Return to Sally Begay's room, obtain a set of vital signs, and conduct a physical exam of her chest and upper extremities. Record your findings in questions 26 and 27 (for Thursday 0800).

26. Below, record your findings from Sally Begay's EPR on Saturday at 1600. (See your answers to question 31 in Lesson 8.) Compare those answers with the findings you recorded during your room visit.

	EPR Data Saturday 1600	Data from Room Visit Thursday 0800
Temperature		
Heart rate		
Blood pressure		
Respiratory rate		
Pain rating, source, characteristics		
Respiratory pattern		
Lung sounds		
Cough		
Sputum		

27. Below, record your answers from question 32 in Lesson 8 (for Saturday 2000). Now compare those findings with the data you obtained during your room visit (Thursday 0800).

	Saturday 2000	Thursday 0800
Pulse oximetry		
Oxygen flow/source		

28. Based on your comparisons in questions 26 and 27, how successful have interventions to improve Sally Begay's chronic bronchitis been to this point? What specific data support your analysis?

29. What further interventions could be implemented to help achieve your desired outcomes?

30. What interventions, if any, should be implemented for Sally Begay with regard to her presumed past exposure to pulmonary tuberculosis?

Complementary Therapies

Reading Assignment: Introduction to Complementary and Alternative Therapies
(Chapter 4)
Patient: Sally Begay, Room 304

This lesson addresses complementary and alternative therapies and their possible application to Sally Begay.

In the Supervisor's Office, sign in to work with Sally Begay for the Tuesday 1100 shift. Go to her room and listen to her responses to the questions in the Value/Belief category of the health history interview.

1. What complementary or alternative therapy does Sally Begay intend to use?

2. If you are unfamiliar with her choice of complementary therapies, how might you get more information?

3. What are some of the varied reactions you might expect to get from Sally Begay or from colleagues in response to your request for information about complementary therapies?

4. Assume that you are Sally Begay's nurse and that you must prepare an interagency report about her to another health care facility. How will you describe her beliefs and choice of complementary therapies?

5. How might the use of humor as a complementary therapy need to be adjusted, given Sally Begay's culture and background? (Review the section on Laughter and Humor in your textbook.)

6. As part of an assessment of complementary therapies, what areas should the nurse explore with Sally Begay?

7. Explain in your own words the difference between *spirituality* and *religion*.

8. What does Sally Begay say is important to her?

9. Develop a plan of care for Sally Begay for the nursing diagnosis Risk for spiritual distress. (Use an NIC manual or any nursing diagnosis textbook for help).

Community-Based Care

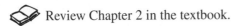 **Reading Assignment:** Community-Based Care (Chapter 2)
Patient: Sally Begay, Room 304

In this lesson, you will consider the community-based care needs of your patient, Sally Begay.

Review Chapter 2 in the textbook.

1. What types of ambulatory care is Sally Begay likely to use after discharge?

2. What are some major responsibilities of the nurse in ambulatory care?

Sign in to work with Sally Begay for the Thursday 1100 shift. Attend the health team meeting in Room 306 and listen to each team member's report on this patient.

3. According to the nurse case manager, what are Sally Begay's two greatest needs for discharge planning purposes.

4. What is the clinical nurse specialist's major concern about Sally Begay's discharge plan?

5. Identify the four concerns that the social worker has about Sally Begay's discharge plan.

6. Are the needs and concerns identified by the health team members appropriate for management by a nurse in ambulatory care?

 Review the community-based care and teaching needed by the patient with COPD and the patient with pneumonia (Chapters 30 and 31 in the textbook).

7. Using the textbook and your answers to questions 3, 4, and 5, complete the chart below.

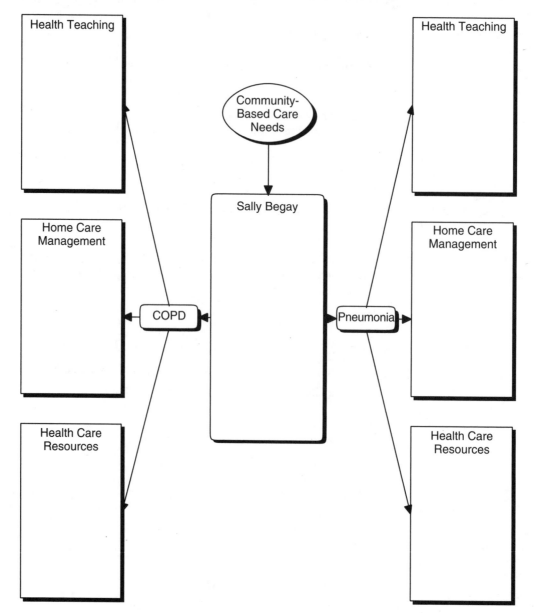

8. List the most important items to include in a plan of care to address Sally Begay's needs in the community. Consider the skilled nursing activities reimbursed by Medicare (discussed in your textbook) as you develop your list.

9. Based on the items you identified for inclusion in a plan of care for Sally Begay in the community, what are some outcome measures that you would want to document?

10. What is the rationale for having a standardized set of patient outcomes (OASIS) in Medicare-funded home health agencies?

14

Evaluation of Care

/OO **Reading Assignment:** Interventions for Clients with Noninfectious Lower Respiratory Problems (Chapter 30)
Interventions for Clients with Infectious Respiratory Problems (Chapter 31)
Patient: Sally Begay, Room 304

Sally Begay, will soon be discharged. As her nurse, it will be your responsibility to make sure that she has all the needed information regarding her immediate care after hospitalization.

1. What information do most patients need upon discharge from the hospital?

2. What information needs to be included in a discharge nurse's note for Sally Begay's medical record?

In the Supervisor's Office, sign in to work with Sally Begay on Thursday at 1100. Go to Room 306 and listen to the report on this patient.

3. The nurse giving report states that Sally Begay has some prescriptions on her chart and a follow-up appointment in 1 week. For which medications would you anticipate that the physician has written prescriptions?

4. What information about the medications should be given to Sally Begay?

 5. Review the evaluation outcomes for COPD and pneumonia (Chapters 30 and 31 in your textbook). In the left column below, list the outcomes suggested for each disease. (You will fill in the remaining columns in question 6.)

Outcomes	Nurses' Notes	Physicians' Notes	EPR
COPD			
Pneumonia			

Now search Sally Begay's EPR, as well as the nurses' notes and physicians' notes in her chart, for evidence of outcome attainment.

6. Document your findings on the chart in question 5. For each outcome you listed, indicate whether or not you found evidence of that outcome being achieved. Next to each outcome, under the corresponding source of data, record a **Y** if you found evidence of outcome attainment or an **N** if you found evidence that the outcome had not been achieved. If the outcome was not mentioned in the data, record **NM**.

7. Review your chart carefully. What outcomes need to be evaluated and noted?

➡ Return to Sally Begay's chart. This time, click on **Health Team** and read the report of each health team member.

8. Now that you have reviewed Sally Begay's chart data and considered the health team members' concerns for her, do you believe any health problem has been overlooked for this patient during this time? Explain.

9. If you answered "yes" to question 8, how might the nurse discharging Sally Begay remedy the oversight you identified?

Ira Bradley

HIV/AIDS

/⟲⟳ **Reading Assignment:** Intervention for Clients with HIV and Other Immunodeficiencies
(Chapter 22)
Patient: Ira Bradley, Room 309

For this lesson, you have been assigned to care for Ira Bradley, a 43-year-old male admitted with late-stage HIV, *Pneumocystis carinii* pneumonia, candidiasis, Kaposi's sarcoma, forehead laceration, and dehydration.

Pathophysiology

 Before you begin working with the patient, review the pathophysiology of HIV in Chapter 22 of your textbook.

1. Briefly explain the difference between primary and secondary immunodeficiencies.

2. Explain why nurses are concerned about patients who are immunodeficient.

111

Review the Centers for Disease Control (CDC) classification scheme for HIV infection in Table 22-2 in your textbook.

3. The CDC considers a person to have acquired immunodeficiency syndrome (AIDS) at the stage of what clinical category of HIV infection?

 Please go to the Supervisor's Office and sign in to work with Ira Bradley for the Tuesday 1100 shift. Open his chart in the Nurses' Station and read the entire Physical & History, including the Emergency Department Report. (Remember to scroll down to read all pages.)

4. Based on your review of Ira Bradley's Physical & History, what is his probable clinical category, according to the CDC classification criteria?

5. What specific data in Ira Bradley's Emergency Department Report and other sections of his Physical & History support your answer to question 4? Record your findings below. If necessary, refer again to Chapter 22 in your textbook to review the CDC criteria for classification in this clinical category.

6. What other diagnostic or laboratory finding supports a medical diagnosis of AIDS?

Etiology

7. Describe the sequence of events from entry of the HIV retrovirus to malfunction of the immune system.

Incidence/Prevalence

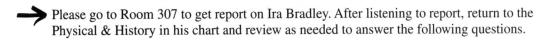 Please go to Room 307 to get report on Ira Bradley. After listening to report, return to the Physical & History in his chart and review as needed to answer the following questions.

8. What risk factors does Ira Bradley have for HIV?

9. Ira Bradley's Physical & History states that the source of his infection is unknown. How important is it to determine the source of his infection at this time?

 10. Identify three specific recommendations for preventing HIV infection among health care workers. Refer to Table 22-5 in your textbook.

Assessment

11. Complete the chart below to illustrate how Ira Bradley's Physical & History assessment findings compare with the expected findings identified in the textbook. Refer to Chart 22-4 for help.

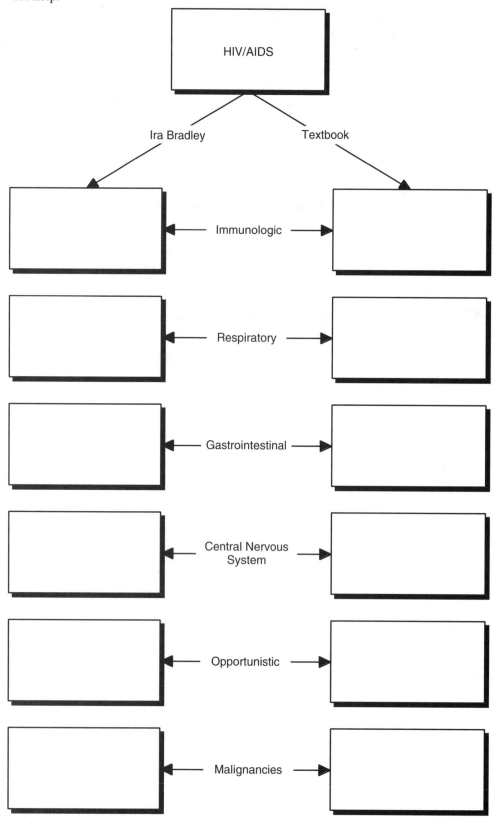

→ 12. Now visit Ira Bradley in his room. Take his vital signs and conduct a complete physical examination. Record your findings below and in the EPR.

Findings

Vital Signs
  Temperature

  Heart rate

  Respiratory rate

  Pulse oximetry

  Blood pressure

  Pain rating, location, characteristics

Head and Neck Examination
  Pupils

  Oral cavity

  Lymph glands

Chest/Upper Extremities
  Chest symmetry

  Heart sounds

  Lung sounds: anterior chest

  Lung sounds: posterior chest

  Tactile fremitus

  Hand strength

Abdomen and Lower Extremities
  Bowel sounds

  Edema

  Foot strength

Now conduct a complete health history interview of Ira Bradley. Listen to his response to questions in all 12 functional health pattern categories.

13. Below, record your findings from each category of Ira Bradley's health history.

Health History Category	Findings
Perception/Self-Concept	
Activity	
Sexuality/Reproductive	
Culture	
Sleep-Rest	
Nutrition-Metabolic	
Role/Relationship	
Health Perception	
Elimination	
Cognitive/Perceptual	
Coping/Stress	
Value/Belief	

Analysis

14. Are there discrepancies between your findings from Ira Bradley's health history interview and the data recorded in the Physical & History in his chart. If so, explain. (Review chart data as necessary.)

15. If you answered "yes" to question 14, what is the most probable reason for the discrepancies between the data you collected and the information recorded by the admitting nurse?

16. Now that you have had a chance to speak with Ira Bradley and his wife during the health history interview, what possible causes can you suggest for his symptoms before admission to the Emergency Department on Sunday?

→ Return to Ira Bradley's chart and locate the physician's admission orders on Sunday.

17. Identify the medications that the physician ordered specifically to combat AIDS. Consult Chart 22-9 in your textbook for help.

18. Identify the major classifications and the specific subclassifications for the drugs you listed in question 17.

19. Are the dosages and times ordered for administration of these drugs consistent with recommendations in your textbook or a drug reference book? Explain.

20. What other subclass of antiretroviral drugs is available?

21. Explain the rationale for highly active antiretroviral therapy (HAART).

22. What are three major disadvantages of HAART?

Planning/Implementation

23. Review the concept map entitled Infection with Human Immunodeficiency Virus in your textbook for suggestions for developing a clinical correlation map. Using the textbook map as an example, develop your own concept map for Ira Bradley on a separate sheet of paper.

24. Based on the data in Ira Bradley's Emergency Department Report, what nursing diagnoses should the admitting nurse have identified for him on Sunday evening? Give your rationale for the selections.

25. The textbook lists nine common nursing diagnoses that should be considered when planning care for a patient with AIDS. Which of these nursing diagnoses are consistent with your assessment of Ira Bradley this morning?

26. In addition to the nursing diagnoses, what collaborative problem is suggested by your analysis of Ira Bradley's data?

27. Prioritize the nursing diagnoses and the collaborative problem you identified in questions 25 and 26 by numbering them from highest to lowest priority. Offer a brief rationale for the order in which you placed them.

28. In the left column below and on the next page, list the nursing diagnoses you prioritized in question 17. (Leave plenty of space between entries.) For each diagnosis, select one or two expected outcomes for Ira Bradley. Next, offer appropriate nursing interventions for the outcomes you identified. (Consult your textbook or an NIC manual for interventions.) Finally, provide rationales to explain how these interventions will help to achieve the expected outcomes.

Nursing Diagnosis/ Collaborative Problem	Expected Outcome(s)	Nursing Interventions	Rationale

Nursing Diagnosis/ Collaborative Problem	Expected Outcome(s)	Nursing Interventions	Rationale

➡ Access Ira Bradley's EPR and locate his data from Sunday at 2400 for each of the vital signs and examination areas listed in question 29 below.

Evaluation

29. Compare the vital signs and physical examination data you obtained from Ira Bradley this morning (see your answer to question 12 of this lesson) with the data recorded in the EPR on Sunday at 2400. (Use **NM** for any findings not recorded on Sunday.)

	EPR Data Sunday 2400	Data from Room Visit Tuesday 0800
Temperature		
Heart rate		
Blood pressure		
Respiratory rate		
Lung sounds		
Pain rating, source, characteristics		
Bowel sounds		
Orientation		

30. Below, record Ira Bradley's oxygen flow, oxygen source, and pulse oximetry readings on Sunday at 2400 from his vital signs summary in the EPR and the results you obtained this morning (Tuesday morning at 0800).

	Sunday 2400	Tuesday 0800
Pulse oximetry		
Oxygen flow/source		

➡ To complete question 31, you will need to review Ira Bradley's I&O and ADL summaries in the EPR, as well as the nurses' notes in his chart.

31. Based on your review of the I&O and nurses' notes, compare Ira Bradley's nutritional intake on Monday at 0800 and Tuesday at 0800. (Use **NM** for any findings not recorded.)

	Monday 0800	Tuesday 0800
Appetite		
Oral fluids		
Weight		

32. Based on your comparisons in questions 30, 31, and 32, how successful have interventions to combat Ira Bradley's chief problems been to this point? What specific data support your analysis?

33. What further interventions could be implemented to help achieve the desired outcomes?

Pain

Reading Assignment: Pain: The Fifth Vital Sign (Chapter 7)
Patient: Ira Bradley, Room 309

Continue working with Ira Bradley, this time focusing on the pain he is experiencing. Remember, he is 43 years old and was admitted with late-stage HIV, *Pneumocystis carinii* pneumonia, candidiasis, Kaposi's sarcoma, forehead laceration, and dehydration.

Before you begin working with the patient, review the pathophysiology of candidiasis in Chapter 22 of your textbook.

1. Given the pathophysiology of candidiasis, what is the most likely source of Ira Bradley's pain?

Please go to the Supervisor's Office and sign in to work with Ira Bradley for the Thursday 1100 shift. In the Nurses' Station, open his chart and review his Physical & History, focusing on data related to his perception of pain. (Remember to scroll down to read all pages.) Then go to the patient's room and obtain a complete set of vital signs. Also observe his health history interview—particularly his responses in the Cognitive-Perceptual category.

2. What specific factors have you learned about Ira Bradley and his history that may influence his perceptions of pain?

3. What type of pain is Ira Bradley probably experiencing?

4. What specific information gathered from Ira Bradley during the health history interview supports your answer to question 3?

Assessment

5. According to the data you have reviewed, how long has Ira Bradley been experiencing his pain?

6. What assessment tool did the nurse use when she asked Ira Bradley to rate his pain during the room visit? See Figure 7-4 in the textbook for help.

7. What other types of pain rating measurement scale might be helpful to use with Ira Bradley?

8. What advantages do the scales you identified in question 7 have compared with the tool the nurse used with Ira Bradley (your answer to question 6)?

Analysis

9. When you were obtaining Ira Bradley's vital signs, did it seem easy or difficult for him to rate the pain sensation he was experiencing?

10. How easy did it seem for him to locate where his pain was occurring?

 11. Review the elements of a complete pain history in your textbook. Based on your reading, how complete do you consider the documentation regarding Ira Bradley's pain? Are precipitating factors, aggravating factors, localization of pain, character and quality of pain, and duration of pain clearly stated? Be sure to check all relevant sources available to you on the CD-ROM before making your assessment.

12. Where on the CD-ROM did you find the information necessary to answer question 11?

Planning/Implementation

13. What nursing diagnoses or collaborative problems would you select for Ira Bradley based on his pain assessment?

14. What outcome measures will indicate success in managing Ira Bradley's pain? Review Evaluation: Outcomes in your textbook or an NOC manual under Comfort Level, Pain Control, Pain: Disruptive Effects, or Pain Level for suggestions.

15. What interventions other than medications may help alleviate Ira Bradley's mouth and throat pain? Review nursing interventions for patients with alterered nutrition in Chapter 22 of your textbook. You may also wish to consult an NIC manual for appropriate interventions.

16. Explain why your selected interventions should help decrease Ira Bradley's pain.

Evaluation

 Access Ira Bradley's EPR, click on **Vital Signs**, and locate the data regarding his pain.

17. Below, record the rating, source, and characteristics of Ira Bradley's pain documented in the EPR on Monday at 1200 and Tuesday at 1200.

	Monday 1200	Tuesday 1200
Pain rating		
Pain source		
Pain characteristics		

18. Based on a comparison of Ira Bradley's pain in question 17, how successful have interventions to combat his pain been to this point?

19. What specific data support your analysis?

20. What further interventions might be implemented to help achieve the desired outcomes?

Cultural Aspects of Care

👓 **Reading Assignment:** Cultural Aspects of Health (Chapter 6)
Patient: Ira Bradley, Room 309

This lesson focuses on the cultural aspects of health and how they affect the care you provide for your patient, Ira Bradley.

💿 Please go to the Supervisor's Office and sign in to work with Ira Bradley for the Thursday 1100 shift. In the Nurses' Station, open his chart and review the Physical & History, scrolling down to read all pages. Go to patient's room and observe the health history interview, especially his responses to questions in the Culture and Value/Belief categories.

1. How does Ira Bradley identify himself?

2. How would you define *middle class professional*? (Hint: Refer to a sociology textbook or try an Internet search using "middle class" and "professional" as key words. Be sure to include the quotation marks since search engines such as Yahoo will then select only site descriptions with those specific terms [i.e., all words in the order specified within a particular set of quotation marks, such as "middle class"]. If you do not use the quotation marks, the search engine will locate site descriptions that may include only one of the terms you specified, as well as sites that include more than one of your key words—but in no particular order.)

3. Does your definition of *middle class professional* seem to match Ira Bradley?

4. What evidence of spirituality did Ira Bradley voice during his health interview?

5. How do you interpret his statement that he is "not very religious"?

6. What questions might you ask to determine whether there are any foods or beverages that Ira Bradley either prefers or considers unacceptable because of his culture?

7. How might your questions be considered inappropriate by Ira Bradley or his family?

8. Use your favorite Internet search engine (if you don't have one, try *http://www.yahoo.com*) and do a search using the key words "Jewish culture." Be sure to include the quotation marks. List some of the websites from your search.

9. List some foods that are strongly identified with Jewish culture. (Even if you are able to answer this on your own, verify your answer by going to one or more of the websites found in your Internet search in question 8. Remember that the weblinks for your textbook will also provide websites on this topic.)

10. Where did you get your information about Jewish foods?

11. How accurate and comprehensive do you think your information source is? On what do you base your opinion?

12. What cultural practice does Ira Bradley plan to use while he is hospitalized?

13. How can a health care institution such as an acute care hospital help Ira Bradley feel more comfortable?

Malnutrition

👓 **Reading Assignment:** Concepts of Inflammation and the Immune Response (Chapter 20)
Interventions for Clients with Connective Tissue Disease
(Chapter 21)
Interventions for Clients with Malnutrition and Obesity
(Chapter 61)

Patient: Ira Bradley, Room 309

In this lesson, you will focus specifically on issues related to malnutrition and its impact on Ira Bradley. As you complete the exercises in this lesson, keep in mind that this patient has late-stage HIV, *Pneumocystis carinii* pneumonia, candidiasis, Kaposi's sarcoma, forehead laceration, and dehydration.

Pathophysiology

 Review the pathophysiology and etiology of nutrition-related immunodeficiencies in Chapter 20 of your textbook.

1. Briefly summarize the association between adequate and balanced nutrition and immune system functioning.

2. How does the association you described in question 1 relate to Ira Bradley?

3. Based on your textbook reading, identify four possible reasons for Ira Bradley's poor nutrition.

Please go to the Supervisor's Office and sign in to work with Ira Bradley for the Thursday 0700 shift. Review the Physical & History section of his chart in the Nurses' Station. (Remember to scroll down to read all pages.)

4. Which, if any, of the reasons for poor nutrition (identified in question 3) does Ira Bradley exhibit?

5. What laboratory values provide monitoring information about nutritional status? (Refer to Chart 22-14 in your textbook for help.)

Assessment

→ Access Ira Bradley's EPR and review his chemistry and hematology data at the time of his admission.

6. Complete the chart below to illustrate how Ira Bradley's laboratory findings on admission compare with the expected findings identified in the textbook for a patient with poor nutrition. In the center boxes, record the normal value ranges for each diagnostic test listed. In the box to the left of each test, record Ira Bradley's results. To the right of each test, indicate the expected findings (from the textbook). Consult Chapter 61, especially Chart 61-5, for help.

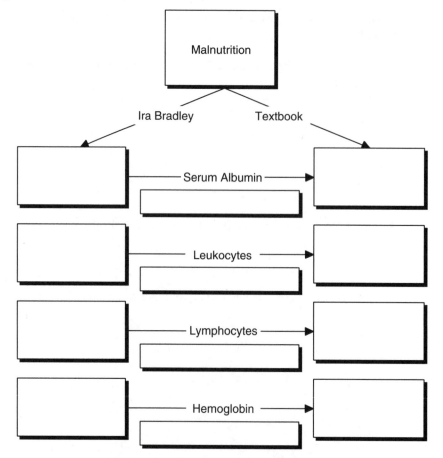

➡️ Review Ira Bradley's Physical & History (in the chart), Admissions Profile (in the EPR), and the health history interview and physical examination (in his room), looking for evidence to support the nursing diagnosis Altered nutrition: less than body requirements.

7. Complete the chart below to illustrate how Ira Bradley's data compare with the expected findings identified in Table 61-4 in your textbook.

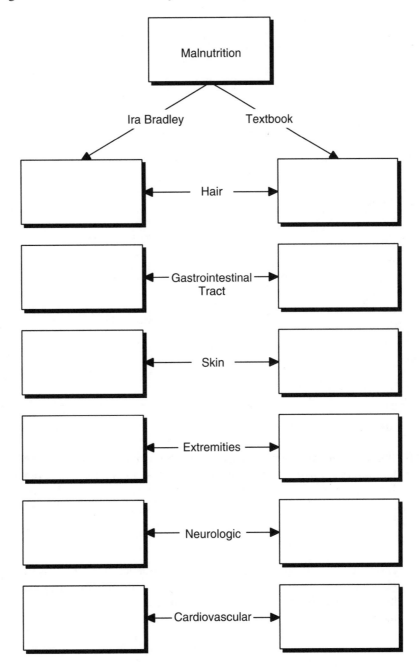

Analysis

8. What are two additional nursing diagnoses or collaborative problems for patients with malnutrition?

9. What data from Ira Bradley's chart and from your physical examination support each diagnosis listed below?

	Chart and/or Physical Examination Data
Impaired skin integrity	
CP: Infection	

Planning

10. In addition to Altered nutrition: less than body requirements, Impaired skin integrity, and CP: Infection, what other nursing diagnosis(es) and/or collaborative problem(s) do Ira Bradley's chart, EPR, and clinical manifestations suggest related to his nutritional status?

11. List below all the nursing diagnoses and/or collaborative problems that have been identified for Ira Bradley based on his clinical manifestations of poor nutrition. Number them from highest to lowest priority and explain your reason for the order in which you prioritized them.

12. In the left column below and on the next page, list the nursing diagnoses you prioritized in question 11. (Leave plenty of space between entries.) For each diagnosis, select one or two expected outcomes for Ira Bradley. Next, offer appropriate nursing interventions for the outcomes. (Consult Chart 61-3 in your textbook or an NIC manual for interventions.) Finally, provide rationales to explain how these interventions will help to achieve the expected outcomes.

Nursing Diagnosis/ Collaborative Problem	Expected Outcome(s)	Nursing Interventions	Rationale

Nursing Diagnosis/ Collaborative Problem	Expected Outcome(s)	Nursing Interventions	Rationale

Evaluation

 Go to Ira Bradley's room and obtain a complete set of vital signs. Then access his EPR and locate the vital signs recorded for him on Saturday at 2400.

13. For each vital sign listed below, record the data documented in the EPR on Sunday at 2400, as well as the findings you just obtained during your assessment in Ira Bradley's room.

	EPR Data Sunday 2400	Data from Room Visit Thursday 0800
Temperature		
Heart rate		
Blood pressure		
Respiratory rate		
Pain rating, source, characteristics		

 Go to the Nurses' Station and open Ira Bradley's chart. In the Emergency Department Report of the Physical & History, note on Sunday at 2400 for data related to oral intake, weight, and appetite. Then access his EPR and review the I&O and ADL summaries for Thursday 0800.

14. Below, record and compare the data you found in the chart for Sunday 2400, in the EPR for Thursday 0800, and in the EPR for Tuesday 0800 (see question 31 in Lesson 15). Use **NM** for any data not recorded.

	Chart Data Sunday 2400	EPR Data Tuesday 0800	EPR Data Thursday 0800
Oral intake			
Weight			
Appetite			

15. Based on your comparisons in questions 13 and 14, how successful have interventions to improve Ira Bradley's undernutrition been to this point? What specific data support your analysis?

16. What further data should have been documented in Ira Bradley's chart and/or EPR for purposes of evaluation?

17. What further interventions could be implemented to help achieve the desired outcomes?

19

End-of-Life Issues

👓 **Reading Assignment:** End-of-Life Care (Chapter 9)
Patient: Ira Bradley, Room 309

Because Ira Bradley has late-stage HIV and is not expected to recover, it is appropriate for you, as his nurse, to address end-of-life issues as you care for him.

📖 Before you begin working with the patient, review Chapter 9 in your textbook.

1. Explain how hospice differs from the care provided to patients expected to recover from illness.

2. According to your textbook, what are the three goals for end-of-life care?

💿 Please go to the Supervisor's Office and sign in to work with Ira Bradley for the Thursday 1100 shift. Visit the patient in his room and listen to his responses to the questions in the health history categories of Coping/Stress and Value/Belief. Also, review the Physical & History in his chart. (Scroll down to read all pages.)

137

3. List the major and secondary symptoms of distress at the end of life in the left column below. (Consult your textbook for help.) In the right column, place an **X** next to the symptoms that Ira Bradley is experiencing at this time.

Symptoms of Distress	Ira Bradley
Major	
Secondary	

4. Does Ira Bradley qualify for hospice care at this time? Explain.

5. Does Ira Bradley's hospital record indicate that he has any form of advance directive, such as a durable power of attorney for health care or living will? If you are uncertain about the differences among advance directives, consult your fundamentals textbook.

6. Why is a durable power of attorney for health care important?

7. How does a durable power of attorney for health care differ from a living will?

8. Explain in your own words the difference between active and passive euthanasia.

9. What does the American Nurses' Association Code of Ethics say about end-of-life issues? In addition to your textbook, you may want to consult the ANA site on the Internet at *http://www.ana.org/* for information.

10. During the health history interview, Ira Bradley says that he is Jewish and is thinking more about his religion these days. What is the general view of the use of "extraordinary" life-prolonging measures among those of the Jewish faith? (Review Table 9-1 in your textbook if you need help.)

11. Using your textbook as a guide, develop a plan of care for the Bradleys using the nursing diagnosis Risk for ineffective family coping. Identify the expected outcome and at least six specific nursing interventions that may be implemented for the patient and family. You may want to consult NOC and NIC manuals for additional information.

12. Ira Bradley's wife, Ann Maine, has expressed dismay at the impact of her husband's illness on the emotional well-being of their children and on the economic well-being of the family. What issues might the hospice agency need to address when Ira Bradley returns home?

LESSON 20

Community Care

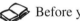 **Reading Assignment:** Community-Based Care (Chapter 2)
Patient: Ira Bradley, Room 309

In this lesson, you will consider the community-based care needs of your patient, Ira Bradley.

Before you begin working with the patient, review Chapter 2 in your textbook.

1. What types of ambulatory care is Ira Bradley likely to use after discharge from the hospital?

2. What are some major responsibilities of the nurse in ambulatory care?

Please go to the Supervisor's Office and sign in to work with Ira Bradley for the Thursday 1100 shift. Listen to the health team report on this patient in Conference Room 2 (Room 308).

3. Identify three principal concerns, for discharge planning purposes, that the nurse case manager expresses in the health team meeting.

141

4. What are the major concerns reported by the clinical nurse specialist related to Ira Bradley's discharge plan?

5. Identify the main concern that the social worker expresses about Ira Bradley's discharge plan.

6. Are the needs identified by the heath team members for Ira Bradley appropriate for management by a nurse in ambulatory care? Explain.

Review the community-based care and teaching needed by the patient with HIV/AIDS in Chapter 22 of your textbook. Use this information to complete the chart on the following page.

7. Based on your textbook reading, as well as your answers to questions 3, 4, and 5 of this lesson, complete the chart below.

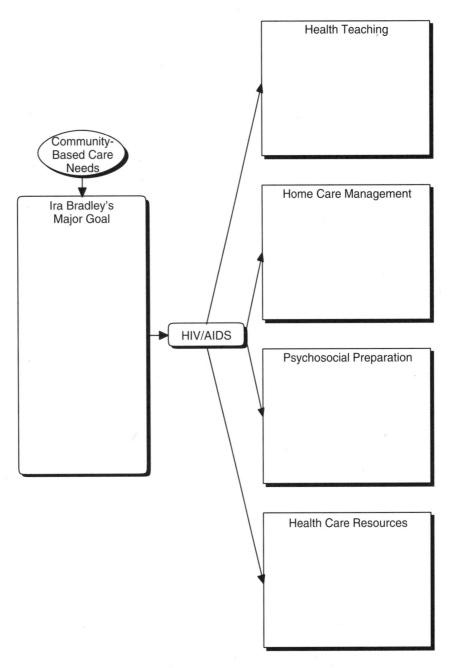

8. What questions should the nurse ask Ira Bradley's wife in regard to the prevention of the spread of HIV infection? (Refer to Chart 22-12 in your textbook.)

9. What information should be included in a discharge plan for Ira Bradley to attempt to prevent future infections? Refer to Chart 22-11 in your textbook. You may also want to consult an NIC manual for other appropriate interventions.

10. Considering the community-based goals you identified for Ira Bradley in question 7, what are some outcome measures that you would want to document?

Evaluation of Care

👓 **Reading Assignment:** Interventions for Clients with HIV and Other Immunodeficiencies (Chapter 22)
Patient: Ira Bradley, Room 309

Ira Bradley will soon be discharged. As his nurse, it will be your responsibility to make sure that
he has all the needed information regarding his immediate care after hospitalization.

1. What are the overall goals for the care of patients with HIV/AIDS?

2. What information needs to be included in a discharge nurse's note for Ira Bradley's medical
record?

In the Supervisor's Office, sign in to work with Ira Bradley on Thursday at 1100. Go to Conference Room 2 (Room 308) and listen to the health team meeting concerning this patient.

3. The clinical nurse specialist and the nurse case manager both express concern about Ira Bradley's medication regimen. Identify at least three critical problems surrounding his medications.

4. What information about the medications should be given to Ira Bradley?

 5. Review the evaluation outcomes for AIDS in Chapter 22 in your textbook. In the left column below, list the outcomes suggested for the disease. (You will fill in the remaining columns in question 6.)

Outcomes	Nurses' Notes	Physicians' Notes	EPR
AIDS			

LESSON 21—EVALUATION OF CARE

IRA BRADLEY

→ Now search Ira Bradley's EPR, as well as the nurses' notes and physicians' notes in his chart, for evidence of outcome attainment.

6. Document your findings on the chart in question 5. For each outcome you listed, indicate whether or not you found evidence of that outcome being achieved. Next to each outcome, under the corresponding source of data, record a **Y** if you found evidence of outcome attainment or an **N** if you found evidence that the outcome had not been achieved. If the outcome was not mentioned in the data, record **NM**.

7. Review your chart carefully. What outcomes need to be evaluated and noted?

→ Return to Ira Bradley's chart. Click on **Health Team** and read the report of each health team member.

8. Now that you have reviewed Ira Bradley's chart data and considered the health team members' concerns for him, do you believe any health problem has been overlooked for this patient during this time? Explain.

9. If you answered "yes" to question 8, how might the nurse discharging Ira Bradley remedy the oversight you identified?

Copyright © 2002 by W.B. Saunders Company. All rights reserved.

● *LESSON* **22** ——————————————————————————————

Fracture

——————————————————————————————

👓 **Reading Assignment:** Interventions for Clients with Musculoskeletal Trauma
(Chapter 52)
Patient: David Ruskin, Room 303

You have been assigned to care for David Ruskin, a 31-year-old African-American male, who was admitted following a bicycle accident. He has a fractured right humerus, scalp laceration, and suspected head trauma.

Pathophysiology

 Before you begin working directly with the patient, review the pathophysiology of fracture in Chapter 52 of your textbook.

1. Identify the criteria by which fractures are classified.

2. Briefly describe the stages of bone healing. For each stage, include the approximate time frame for the healing process in young adults.

Please go to the Supervisor's Office and sign in to work with David Ruskin for the Tuesday 0700 shift. Then go to the Nurses' Lounge (Room 306) and listen to the change-of-shift report on this patient. Next, access the EPR in the Nurses' Station and review his Admissions Profile. Also review the Physical & History in his chart. (Scroll down to read all pages.)

3. Based on what you learned from the change-of-shift report and your review of David Ruskin's chart and Admissions Profile, did you notice any discrepancies between the two sources of data? If so, explain.

4. If you answered "yes" to question 3, does the discrepancy make a significant difference in planning nursing care for David Ruskin? Explain.

5. How can you verify which of the two sources of data is correct?

Incidence/Prevalence

 6. Compare David Ruskin's injuries with the risk factors for fracture identified in your textbook. Does he have a typical history for his injuries? Explain

7. Identify the most common bones fractured by young adults.

Assessment

8. Complete the chart below to illustrate how David Ruskin's Admissions Profile and Physical & History compare with the expected findings for fractured humerus identified in your textbook.

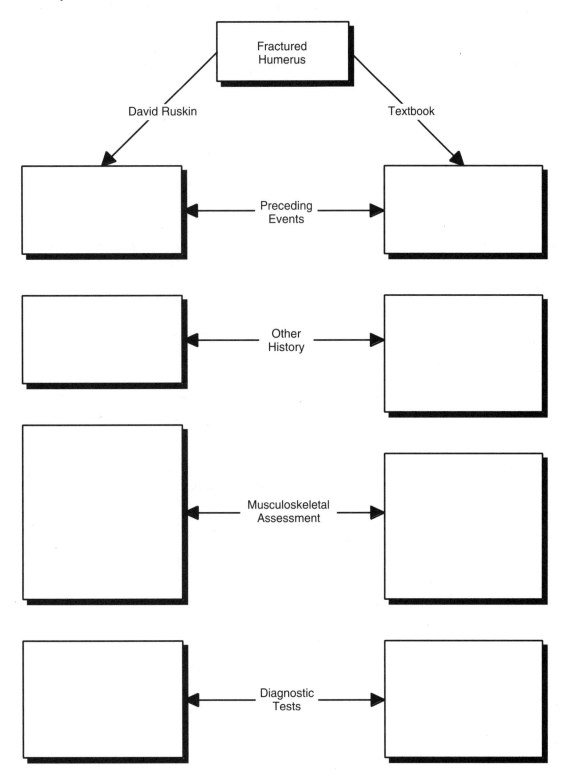

Go to David Ruskin's room and obtain the rating and location of his pain. (Click on **Vital Signs**, then on **Pain**.) Now compare these findings with the pain he was experiencing on admission. To do this, access his EPR and find data related to his pain in the vital signs summary for Sunday at 2000.

9. Record your findings related to David Ruskin's pain below. If a finding is not mentioned in the patient's EPR data, record **NM**.

	EPR Data Sunday 2000	Data from Room Visit Tuesday 0700
Pain rating		
Pain location		

Go to David Ruskin's chart in the Nurses' Station. Click on **Nurses' Notes** and read the notes for Sunday at 2030 and Monday at 1615. Then check the EPR for any relevant related data recorded for these same days.

10. Based on your review, do you believe there are any findings missing from either the nurses' notes or the EPR? What additional data would you like to see documented?

Find data in David Ruskin's chart concerning x-rays taken on admission. (Look in his Emergency Department Report and in the diagnostics section.)

11. Are the findings from David Ruskin's admitting x-ray series consistent with the medical diagnosis of a fractured right humerus? Explain. What type of fracture is reported in his chart, if any?

→ Go to David Ruskin's room and obtain a complete set of vital signs. Also conduct a physical examination of his chest and upper extremities. Then access his EPR and review any data necessary to complete question 12.

12. Below, record the vital signs and physical examination findings from your room visit with David Ruskin. (Document your findings in the EPR as well. If you cannot remember how to record data in the EPR, consult the Getting Started section of this workbook.)

Tuesday 0800 Findings

Respiratory rate

Heart rate

Temperature

Blood pressure

Pulse oximetry

Oxygen source

Pain rating, location

Chest expansion

Respiratory pattern

Lung fields

Cough

Sputum

Radial pulses

Sensory perception

Capillary refill

13. Based on your observation of David Ruskin's physical examination of the chest and upper extremities, provide a critique of the auscultation technique used by his nurse.

 14. Considering the injuries that David Ruskin sustained, are the data you collected about his respiratory status consistent with the expected findings identified by your textbook? Explain.

15. The pulse oximeter was placed on David Ruskin's right index finger when his vital signs were taken. What effect, if any, could this have on the accuracy of the pulse oximetry reading?

 16. Below, identify the complications that commonly occur with fractures and describe the clinical manifestations of each complication. Consult your textbook if you need help.

Complication	Clinical Manifestation

Analysis

17. What are three common nursing diagnoses for patients with a fracture?

18. In the left column below, list the three nursing diagnoses you identified in question 17. For each diagnosis, identify supporting evidence you found during your room visit with David Ruskin and from your review of his chart and EPR data.

Nursing Diagnosis	Data from Room Visit	EPR and/or Chart Data

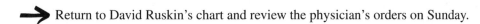 Return to David Ruskin's chart and review the physician's orders on Sunday.

19. Identify the medication that the physician ordered specifically to treat infection.

20. Identify the classification and subclassification of the drug ordered prophylactically for David Ruskin.

21. Are the dosage and time ordered for administration of this drug consistent with recommendations in your textbook or a drug reference book?

22. What is the drug classification for ketorolac? For what adverse effects of this drug should the nurse monitor David Ruskin? Consult a pharmacology textbook if necessary.

Planning/Implementation

23. On a separate sheet of paper, develop a clinical correlation map for David Ruskin. Use the textbook examples in Chapter 52 for ideas. Be sure to identify the patient's clinical manifestations and include potential complications of fractures. Use different colored pens or pencils for your map. A concept map is a working tool that grows as information is added. Neatness and artistic ability are not the primary objectives when developing a concept map.

24. List and prioritize the five most important nursing diagnoses or collaborative problems you have identified for David Ruskin. Number them from highest to lowest priority. Provide a rationale for the order in which you placed them.

25. In the left column below and on the next page, list the nursing diagnoses and/or collaborative problems you prioritized in question 24. (Use both pages and leave plenty of space between entries.) For each nursing diagnosis you identified, select one or two expected outcomes for David Ruskin. Refer to Evaluation: Outcomes in your textbook or an NOC manual for help. Next, provide appropriate nursing interventions for the outcomes you listed. Refer to an NIC manual or your textbook for interventions. Finally, offer rationales to explain how these interventions will help to achieve the expected outcomes.

Nursing Diagnosis/ Collaborative Problem	Expected Outcome(s)	Nursing Interventions	Rationale

Nursing Diagnosis/ Collaborative Problem	Expected Outcome(s)	Nursing Interventions	Rationale

➤ Your next task is to evaluate David Ruskin's progress since his admission on Sunday. Start by accessing his EPR and reviewing his vital signs and assessment data on Sunday at 2000.

Evaluation

26. In the chart below, compare the data you obtained in David Ruskin's room earlier in this lesson (see question 12) with the findings recorded in the EPR on Sunday at 2000.

	EPR Data Sunday 2000	Data from Room Visit Tuesday 0800
Temperature		
Heart rate		
Blood pressure		
Respiratory rate		
Pain rating, location, characteristics		
Respiratory pattern		
Lung sounds		
Cough		
Sputum		

➤ While still in the vital signs summary in the EPR, locate David Ruskin's pulse oximetry and oxygen source data for Sunday at 2000.

27. Below, compare the data you obtained from the EPR with your findings this morning in David Ruskin's room (see question 12 of this lesson).

	EPR Data Sunday 2000	Data from Room Visit Tuesday 0800
Pulse oximetry		
Oxygen source		

28. Below, record David Ruskin's WBC readings on Saturday 2000 and Tuesday 0800. To find these readings, click on **Hematology** in the EPR.

	Saturday 2000	Tuesday 0800
WBC		

29. Based on your comparisons in questions 26, 27, and 28, how successful have interventions to prevent common postoperative complications of David Ruskin's fracture been to this point? What specific data support your analysis?

Traumatic Brain Injury

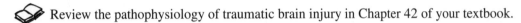 **Reading Assignment:** Interventions for Critically Ill Clients with Neurologic Problems
(Chapter 45)
Patient: David Ruskin, Room 303

In this lesson, you will review issues related to traumatic brain injury and apply what you have
learned to the case of David Ruskin.

Pathophysiology

Review the pathophysiology of traumatic brain injury in Chapter 42 of your textbook.

Sign in to work with David Ruskin on Tuesday at 1100. In the Nurses' Station, open his chart
and review the entire Physical & History, including the Emergency Department Report.
(Remember to scroll down to read all pages.)

1. Based on his Emergency Department Report, what type of traumatic brain injury has David
Ruskin experienced?

2. What type of force did David Ruskin probably experience to his head?

3. The Emergency Department physician ordered a CT scan of David Ruskin's head. What
was the probable purpose for the procedure?

Incidence/Prevalence

 4. How well does David Ruskin match the profile for the individual experiencing traumatic brain injury? Explain. Consult your textbook for help.

Assessment

5. What data should the nurse in the Emergency Department obtain from David Ruskin?

Analysis

6. What was David Ruskin's first recorded Glasgow Coma Scale rating? What does this score and his history indicate about the extent of his traumatic brain injury?

7. Based on your understanding of the extent of David Ruskin's traumatic brain injury, what are some of the possible implications concerning his memory and his behavior?

Planning/Implementation

8. What nursing diagnosis or collaborative problem would you select for David Ruskin based on the assessment data regarding his traumatic brain injury?

→ Go to David Ruskin's room and conduct a physical examination of the head and neck. Then review the Physical & History in his chart as needed to complete question 9.

9. In the left column below, record your nursing diagnosis from question 8. Then list data from the chart and from your interview with David Ruskin that support that diagnosis. Identify where you found your answers.

Nursing Diagnosis	Physical Exam Data	Chart Data

10. In the left column below, write the nursing diagnosis you identified in question 8. Then select one or two expected outcomes for David Ruskin. Next, offer appropriate nursing interventions for the outcomes you identified. (Consult your textbook or an NIC manual for interventions.) Finally, provide rationales to explain how these interventions will help to achieve the expected outcomes.

Nursing Diagnosis	Expected Outcome(s)	Nursing Interventions	Rationale

11. Which of the nursing interventions you identified could be safely delegated to unlicensed personnel? Explain.

Evaluation

 Go to David Ruskin's room and conduct a physical examination of the head and neck and chest/upper extremities. Record your findings for each of the clinical markers listed in question 12 below. After you have finished, return to the Physical & History in his chart and locate data for these same markers recorded on Sunday at 1700.

 12. Below, record your findings from the chart and from your room visit for each physical examination area listed. Review Figure 41-14 in your textbook for information about the Glasgow Coma Scale.

	Chart Data Sunday 1700	Data from Room Visit Tuesday 1100
Pupils		
Orientation		
Nares		
Hand strength		
Glasgow Coma Scale		

13. Based on your comparison of David Ruskin's clinical markers for traumatic brain injury in question 12, would you stop surveillance for traumatic brain injury? Explain.

14. What information about his head injury should be given to David Ruskin and his wife before he goes home?

Cultural Aspects of Care

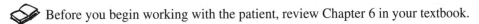 **Reading Assignment:** Cultural Aspects of Care (Chapter 6)
Patient: David Ruskin, Room 303

Continue to care for David Ruskin, this time focusing on the cultural factors that affect his health and the care you give him.

Before you begin working with the patient, review Chapter 6 in your textbook.

Please go to the Supervisor's Office and sign in to work with David Ruskin for the Tuesday 1100 shift. Access the EPR and review his Admissions Profile. Then go to his room and observe the health history interview, focusing particularly on the categories of Culture and Value/Belief.

1. How does David Ruskin identify himself?

2. How did he respond to a question about spirituality during his health interview?

3. How do you describe the difference between the terms *spirituality* and *religion*?

4. David Ruskin states that he is ethnically African-American but adds that he is an "Army brat" and feels that he is a member of several different cultures. What is an "Army brat," and how might this have contributed to the patient's sense of being multicultural?

5. David Ruskin states that English is his preferred language but that he also speaks Spanish and French. Explain how his language acquisition relates to his other interests?

6. When asked about how his values and beliefs guide his decision making, David Ruskin states that he is a pragmatist, and then hesitates and says that he does not understand the question and does not know how to answer it. How could you reframe the question? Consult the section in your textbook on performing a cultural assessment for ideas. Other resources are available on the Internet (try *http://www.wbsaunders.com/SIMON/Iggy/*).

7. David Ruskin states that he feels it is important that he create better opportunities for all people, especially now that he is about to become a father. How does he describe his role in his family?

8. Do an Internet search using "education statistics" and further modify your search using "Master's degree" as keywords. Go to one or more of the websites from your search and review any information concerning the typical profile of graduate students, as well as any characteristics that apply specifically to David Ruskin, such as age, field of study, race, and gender. Remember, you can also find websites on this topic by going to the weblinks for your textbook. How closely do your observations of David Ruskin and his description of himself match your findings about graduate students?

9. Do you think the information source(s) you used to answer question 8 is (are) accurate? Why?

10. How can a health care institution such as an acute care hospital help David Ruskin feel more comfortable?

Pulmonary Embolism and Adult Respiratory Distress Syndrome

 Reading Assignment: Interventions for Critically Ill Clients with Respiratory Problems
(Chapter 32)

Patient: David Ruskin, Room 303

For this lesson, you will focus on pulmonary embolism and adult respiratory distress syndrome and their potential impact on the health of your patient, David Ruskin, a 31-year-old African-American male, who was admitted following a bicycle accident. He has a fractured right humerus, scalp laceration, and suspected head trauma.

Pathophysiology

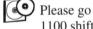 Before you begin working with the patient, review the pathophysiology, etiology, and incidence/prevalence of pulmonary embolism (PE) and adult respiratory distress syndrome (ARDS) in Chapter 32 in your textbook.

Please go to the Supervisor's Office and sign in to work with David Ruskin for the Thursday 1100 shift. Open his chart in the Nurses' Station and review the Physical & History. (Scroll down to read all pages.) Then go to the patient's room and obtain a full set of vital signs.

1. During her morning assessment, the unit nurse asks David Ruskin to rate his pain. How should the pain rating scale be described to him?

2. David Ruskin tells the nurse his pain is located in his chest and is worse when he breathes. What other questions about his pain should the nurse ask?

171

3. How easy do you think it is for David Ruskin to locate where his pain is occurring?

4. Briefly summarize the major pathologic changes that occur in the lung with pulmonary embolism.

5. What is the most common cause for pulmonary embolism?

6. Which of the two graphics below best represents how pulmonary embolism and fat embolism syndrome are related?

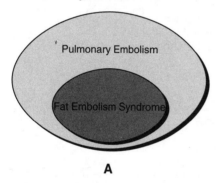

A

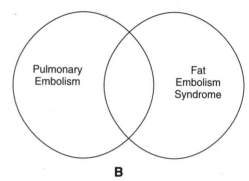

B

Review data in David Ruskin's chart and his EPR as needed to answer the following questions.

7. What assessment data support the medical diagnosis of pulmonary embolism for David Ruskin?

8. Briefly summarize the major pathologic changes that occur in the lung with adult respiratory distress syndrome.

9. What assessment data support the medical diagnosis of adult respiratory distress syndrome for David Ruskin?

Incidence/Prevalence

10. Which, if any, of the causes for pulmonary embolism does David Ruskin have?

11. Compare David Ruskin's risk factors for adult respiratory distress syndrome with those identified in Chapter 32 of your textbook. Which risk factors does he have?

Assessment

➤ Return to David Ruskin's chart and review the diagnostics section.

12. David Ruskin's radiologic report contains information needed to analyze his complaint of chest pain. What information in the radiologic report on Sunday at 1600 should be considered?

13. Complete the chart below to illustrate how David Ruskin's laboratory and radiographic findings on Thursday at 1600 compare with the expected findings identified in your textbook for a patient with either pulmonary embolism or adult respiratory distress syndrome. Refer to Chapter 32 in your textbook for help.

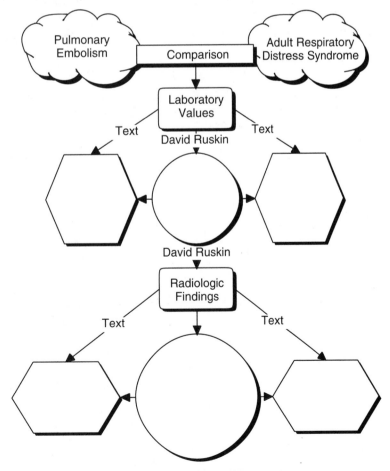

Analysis

14. Complete the Venn comparison diagram on the right below to compare the symptoms of pulmonary embolism, fat embolism syndrome, and adult respiratory distress syndrome. Refer to discussions on clinical manifestations in your textbook.

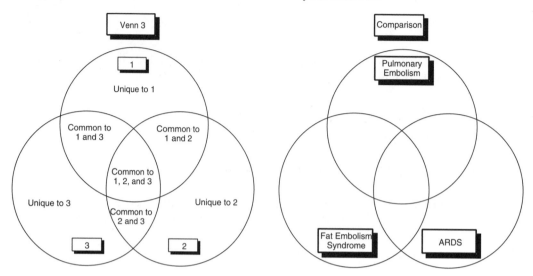

   a. Identify the clinical manifestations that all three respiratory illnesses share.

   b. Identify the clinical manifestations that are the same for pulmonary embolism and fat embolism syndrome.

15. Based on the comparison Venn diagram, what diagnostic findings obtained through physical examination and test results might help differentiate among the three pathologies?

   Physical examination:

   Laboratory/radiologic tests:

16. Considering the pathologic processes, what are two priority nursing diagnoses for patients with possible pulmonary embolism or adult respiratory distress syndrome?

→ Review David Ruskin's chart, EPR data, health history interview, and physical examination as needed to answer the following questions.

17. Listed below are two possible nursing diagnoses for David Ruskin. What data from his chart, EPR, or your room visit support each diagnosis listed?

Nursing Diagnosis	Data from Room Visit	Chart and/or EPR Data
Ineffective tissue perfusion: cardiopulmonary		
Impaired gas exchange		

18. Based on your analysis, would you use the diagnoses listed in question 17, modify them, or select different diagnoses for David Ruskin? Please explain what you would do and why.

Planning

19. What other respiratory nursing diagnosis is suggested by David Ruskin's clinical manifestations?

20. Prioritize the nursing diagnoses you identified for David Ruskin in questions 18 and 19. Number them from highest to lowest priority. Provide a brief rationale for the order in which you placed them.

21. in the left column below, list the nursing diagnoses you prioritized in question 20. For each diagnosis, write one or two expected outcomes. Next, identify appropriate nursing interventions for each outcome. Refer to your textbook or an NIC manual for interventions. Finally, provide rationales to explain how these interventions will help to achieve the expected outcomes.

Nursing Diagnosis	Expected Outcome(s)	Nursing Interventions	Rationale

Evaluation

 Return to David Ruskin's room and obtain the vital signs and physical examination data listed in questions 22 and 23 below. Then find the same data for Sunday at 2400 by checking his vital signs and assessment summaries in the EPR.

22. For each vital sign and physical examination area listed below, record your findings from David Ruskin's EPR and from your room visit.

	EPR Data Sunday 2400	Data from Room Visit Thursday 1100
Heart rate		
Respiratory rate		
Pain rating, source, characteristics		
Respiratory pattern		
Lung fields		
Chest expansion		

23. Below, compare David Ruskin's pulse oximetry readings and his oxygen sources on Sunday and Thursday.

	EPR Data Sunday 2000	Data from Room Visit Thursday 1100
Pulse oximetry		
Oxygen source		

24. Based on your comparisons in questions 22 and 23, how successful have interventions to prevent David Ruskin's pulmonary complications been to this point? What specific data support your analysis?

LESSON 26

Case Management

 Reading Assignment: Introduction to Managed Care and Case Management (Chapter 3)
Patient: David Ruskin, Room 303

This lesson gives you the opportunity to consider issues of case management as they apply to your patient, David Ruskin.

Review Chapter 3 in your textbook.

In the Supervisor's Office, sign in to work with David Ruskin on Thursday at 1100. Access and review any data necessary to complete the questions in this lesson.

1. On Wednesday at 0630, David Ruskin's physician wrote the medical order "Case management to see patient." Using your textbook as a guide, explain the purpose of case management.

2. Why do you think the physician wanted a case manager to see the patient?

3. What duties of the case manager would benefit David Ruskin at this time?

179

4. Identify some likely health care team members with whom the case manager will need to coordinate care.

5. Would the case manager working with David Ruskin more likely be an internal case manager or an external case manager? Explain your decision.

6. Under what medical circumstances might David Ruskin qualify for an external case manager who is working with disease state management? Consider his possible central nervous system and respiratory difficulties in your answer.

7. Describe a clinical pathway. You can find information about clinical pathways on the Simon site (*http://www.wbsaunders.com/SIMON/Iggy/*). Also see examples in your textbook.

8. On which clinical pathway(s) might David Ruskin have been placed?

9. Discuss how this patient might benefit from the use of a clinical pathway.

LESSON 27 ————————————

Community Care

————————————————————————

 Reading Assignment: Community-Based Care (Chapter 2)
Patient: David Ruskin, Room 303

Once again, you have been assigned to care for David Ruskin. In this lesson, you will focus on his community-based care needs.

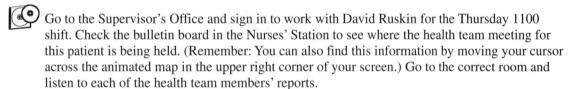 Review Chapter 2 in your textbook.

Go to the Supervisor's Office and sign in to work with David Ruskin for the Thursday 1100 shift. Check the bulletin board in the Nurses' Station to see where the health team meeting for this patient is being held. (Remember: You can also find this information by moving your cursor across the animated map in the upper right corner of your screen.) Go to the correct room and listen to each of the health team members' reports.

1. What type of ambulatory care is David Ruskin likely to use after discharge from the hospital?

2. What are some major responsibilities of the nurse in ambulatory care?

3. Identify the two greatest needs related to discharge planning that the nurse case manager reports in the team meeting.

4. Identify the major concern voiced by the clinical nurse specialist related to David Ruskin's discharge plan.

5. Identify the main concerns that the social worker has for his discharge plan.

6. Are the health care needs identified for David Ruskin by the heath team members appropriate for management by a nurse in ambulatory care? Explain.

 Review the community-based care and teaching necessary for patients with a fracture as discussed in Chapter 52 of your textbook.

7. Based on your textbook reading and your answers to questions 3, 4, and 5, complete the following chart addressing David Ruskin's community-based care needs.

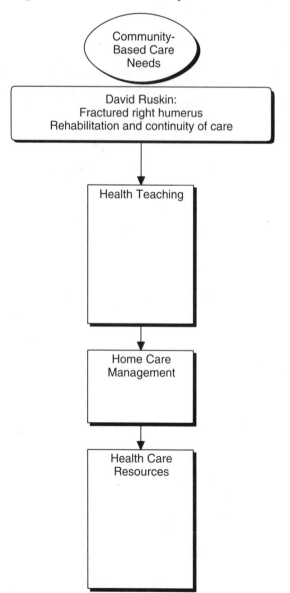

8. Assuming that a home care nurse will make one visit, list the most important items to include in a plan of care to address David Ruskin's needs in the community. Consider the skilled nursing activities reimbursed by Medicare as you develop your list. Consult your textbook for Medicare reimbursements.

9. Based on the items you included in your answer to question 8 for David Ruskin, what outcome measures would you want to document?

LESSON 28

Evaluation of Care

 Reading Assignment: Interventions for Clients with Musculoskeletal Problems
(Chapter 52)
Patient: David Ruskin, Room 303

Your patient, David Ruskin, will soon be discharged. As his nurse, it will be your responsibility to make sure that he has all the needed information regarding his immediate care after hospitalization. Remember that he is 31 years old and was admitted following a bicycle accident in which he suffered a fractured right humerus, scalp laceration, and suspected head trauma.

1. What information do most patients need upon discharge from the hospital?

2. What information needs to be included in a discharge nurse's note for David Ruskin's medical record?

187

3. What information about medications should be given to David Ruskin?

 4. Review the evaluation outcomes for fractures in Chapter 52 of your textbook. In the left column below, list the expected outcomes suggested. (You will fill in the other columns in question 5.)

Expected Outcomes	Nurses' Notes	Physicians' Notes	EPR

Fractures

 In the Supervisor's Office, sign in to care for David Ruskin on Thursday at 1100. Go to the Nurses' Station and open his chart. Review the nurses' notes and physicians' notes, looking for evidence that indicates whether or not the outcomes for fracture suggested by your textbook have been achieved in this patient's case. Then access the EPR and search for the same evidence in his data summaries.

5. Record your findings on the chart in question 4 above. Next to each outcome, under the corresponding CD source of data, record a **Y** if you found evidence of outcome attainment, record an **N** if you found evidence that the outcome had not been achieved, and record **NM** if the outcome was not mentioned.

6. Based on your chart in question 4, what outcomes need to be evaluated and noted?

7. There are few physicians' notes, although the clinical record indicates that a physician wrote medical treatment orders for David Ruskin on a daily basis. What are some of the legal implications of this observation? You made need to review the requirements for documentation in a fundamentals textbook.

➡ Check the bulletin board in the Nurses' Station or move your cursor across the animated map to see where the health team meeting for David Ruskin is being held. Go to that room and listen to each member's report.

8. Now that you have reviewed the data documented in David Ruskin's chart and EPR and listened to the health team members' concerns, what health problem has been overlooked during his hospitalization?

9. Based on what you learned from the health team meeting, which members of the health team will need to see David Ruskin most frequently during his recovery period?

Andrea Wang

LESSON **29** ——————————————————————

Spinal Cord Injury

———————————————————————————————————————

    Reading Assignment: Intervention for Clients with Problems of the Central Nervous System: The Spinal Cord (Chapter 43)

    Patient: Andrea Wang, Room 310

You have been assigned to care for Andrea Wang, a 20-year-old Asian-American female, who was admitted following a diving accident. She has a burst fracture at T6 and a partial transection of the spinal cord. She has been admitted to the medical-surgical unit after a week in ICU.

Pathophysiology

Before you begin, review the pathophysiology of spinal cord injury (SCI) in Chapter 43 of your textbook.

    1. Identify and briefly describe four mechanisms that may result in spinal cord injury. Include an example of how each mechanism may occur.

Sign in to care for Andrea Wang on Tuesday at 0700. Open her chart and review the Physical & History, including the Emergency Department Record. Click on **Diagnostics** and review the radiology reports. Close the chart and access Andrea Wang's EPR. Review any data relevant to spinal cord injury recorded at the time of her admission.

2. Of the mechanisms you identified in question 1, which type of force did Andrea Wang most likely experience? Explain your answer.

3. Review Figure 43-5 in your textbook. Given the descriptions of the injury to Andrea Wang's spine in her radiology reports, what assessments would you want to make?

4. Describe anterior cord syndrome and identify some assessment data that might be expected with this condition.

 5. Andrea Wang sustained her SCI during swimming practice when she flipped off a diving board and landed on the concrete pool edge. How does the description of the cause of her injury compare with the common causes of SCI?

Incidence/Prevalence

6. After reading Andrea Wang's Physical & History, compare her risk factors for SCI with those identified in your textbook. Which risk factors does she have?

Assessment

7. Complete the chart below to illustrate how Andrea Wang's chart and EPR findings compare with the expected findings identified in the textbook.

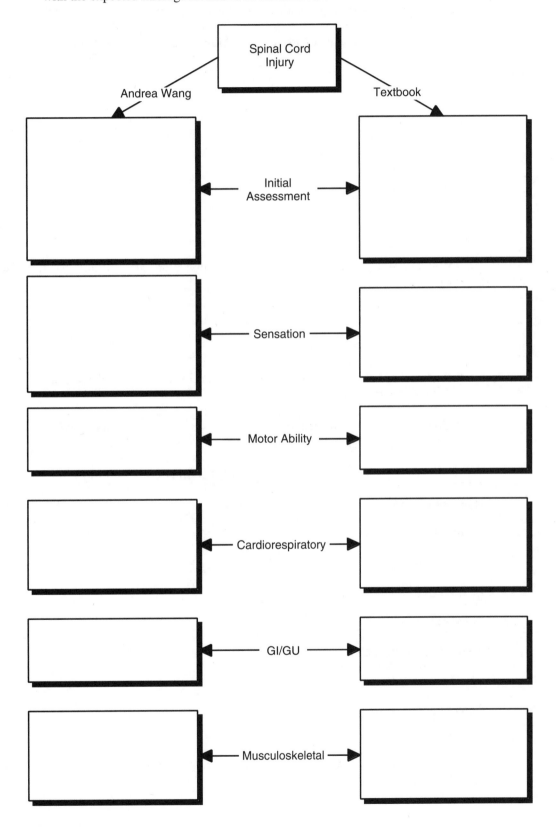

→ Access and review Andrea Wang's chart and EPR as needed to answer question 8.

8. Andrea Wang was admitted to the Emergency Department on Sunday at 1230. Based on her chart and EPR data for each of the times listed below, record her pulse oximetry, respiratory rate and pattern, and oxygen source. Also include the amount of supplemental oxygen she was using, if any.

	Sun 1230	**Mon 1200**	**Mon 2400**	**Tues 0800**
Pulse oximetry				
Respiratory rate				
Respiratory pattern				
Oxygen source				

9. Do Andrea Wang's vital signs recorded in question 8 indicate that she is having difficulty maintaining adequate oxygen? Explain.

→ Go to Andrea Wang's room, take her vital signs, and conduct a physical examination of her chest and upper extremities.

10. Below, record the data related to respiratory status you obtained during your room visit with Andrea Wang. Document your findings in the EPR as well.

Tuesday 0800 Findings

Respiratory rate

Heart rate

Temperature

Blood pressure

Pulse oximetry

Pain rating, source, characteristics

Chest expansion

Respiratory pattern

Lung fields

11. Are the data you collected in question 10 consistent with the textbook?

→ Now conduct a physical examination of Andrea Wang's abdomen and lower extremities.

12. Record your findings below and on the EPR.

Tuesday 0800 Findings

Bowel sounds on
    palpation

Dorsalis pedis pulses

Posterior tibial pulses

Capillary refill

Skin temperature/color

Catheter tubing

Analysis

13. What further assessments should be made at this time? Why?

 14. What two common nursing diagnoses for patients with SCI apply to Andrea Wang? Consult your textbook for common diagnoses.

15. In the left column below, list the two nursing diagnoses you identified in question 14. For each diagnosis, identify supporting data from Andrea Wang's chart and from your physical examination and vital signs finding.

Nursing Diagnosis	Data from Physical Examination and Vital Signs	Data from Patient's Chart

16. A common collaborative problem with spinal cord injury is CP: Potential for deep vein thrombosis. What risk factors does Andrea Wang have that increase her risk for DVT? (See your textbook if you need help.)

17. Chapter 43 in your textbook lists seven other nursing diagnoses that should be considered when planning care for a patient with SCI. Which of these additional nursing diagnoses are consistent with your assessment of Andrea Wang?

In Andrea Wang's chart, locate and review the physician's postoperative orders for Sunday.

18. Identify the medications or other measures that the physician ordered specifically to prevent common complications of SCI. (Consult your textbook for help.)

19. What are the recommended dosages and times for administration of these drugs, according to a drug reference book or pharmacology textbook?

20. Are the dosages and times ordered by Andrea Wang's physician consistent with the recommendations you identified in question 19? If not, explain.

21. Which drugs ordered by the physician should help to reduce Andrea Wang's pain level? Explain how each drug will accomplish this goal.

Planning/Implementation

 22. Refer to any of the concept maps in your textbook for suggestions for developing a clinical correlation map. On a separate sheet of paper, develop your own clinical correlation map for Andrea Wang. Use different colored pens and pencils for your map.

23. List below all of the potential nursing diagnoses and collaborative problems that have been identified or suggested for Andrea Wang in questions 14 through 17. Number them from highest to lowest priority and provide a rationale for the order in which you prioritized them.

24. In the left column below, list the first three nursing diagnoses and/or collaborative problems you prioritized in question 23. (Leave plenty of space between entries.) For each diagnosis or collaborative problem, select one or two expected outcomes for Andrea Wang. Refer to Evaluation: Outcomes in the textbook or an NOC manual for help. Next, provide appropriate nursing interventions for the outcomes you identified. Consult your textbook or an NIC manual for interventions. Finally, offer rationales to explain how these interventions will help to achieve the expected outcomes.

Nursing Diagnosis/ Collaborative Problem	Expected Outcome(s)	Nursing Interventions	Rationale

Access Andrea Wang's EPR and review her vital signs and assessment data for Sunday at 1600.

Evaluation

25. Below, record your findings from the EPR for each of the vital signs and physical examination areas listed. Also record the data you obtained earlier in Andrea Wang's room (see question 10 of this lesson). You will need to return to her room to obtain findings for the last three areas since they were not taken earlier.

	EPR Data Sunday 1600	Data from Room Visit Tuesday 0800
Temperature		
Heart rate		
Blood pressure		
Respiratory rate		
Pain rating, source, characteristics		
Respiratory pattern		
Lung sounds		
Sensation/motion		
Bowel sounds		
GU		

26. Based on your comparisons in question 25, how successful have interventions to safeguard Andrea Wang's status and begin restoring her to independent function been to this point? What specific data support your analysis?

27. What further interventions could be implemented to help achieve your desired outcomes?

Autonomic Dysreflexia and Urinary Retention

 Reading Assignment: Interventions for Clients with Problems of the Nervous System: The Spinal Cord (Chapter 43)
Patient: Andrea Wang, Room 310

In this lesson, you will focus specifically on issues related to autonomic dysreflexia and urinary retention and their impact on Andrea Wang.

Pathophysiology

Review the pathophysiology of autonomic dysreflexia and urinary retention in Chapter 43 of your textbook.

1. Draw a flow chart or other diagram to illustrates the sequence of events causing spinal shock. You may need to refer to Chapter 37 in your textbook for further information about neural-induced distributive shock.

Please go to the Supervisor's Office and sign in to work with Andrea Wang for the Friday 1100 shift. Open her chart in the Nurses' Station and review the entire Physical & History, including the Emergency Department Record. (Remember to scroll down to read all pages.) Also review the nurses' notes and the health team reports.

2. Based on your review of the Emergency Department Record, what were Andrea Wang's vital signs upon admission? Record your findings below.

Admission Findings

Temperature

Heart rate

Blood pressure

Respiratory rate

3. What additional clinical manifestations point to spinal shock?

4. Draw a flow chart or diagram to show the sequence of events causing autonomic dysreflexia. You may need to refer to Chapters 41 and 69 in your textbook for further information about autonomic nervous system function and urinary bladder function.

5. Do you believe Andrea Wang needs to be monitored for AD at this time? Explain.

Assessment

→ Access Andrea Wang's EPR and review any data relevant to spinal shock recorded at the time of her admission.

6. Complete the chart below to illustrate how Andrea Wang's assessment findings on admission compare with the expected findings identified in the textbook for a patient with spinal shock. In the boxes on the left, record her results for each assessment area. To the right, indicate the expected findings (from the textbook).

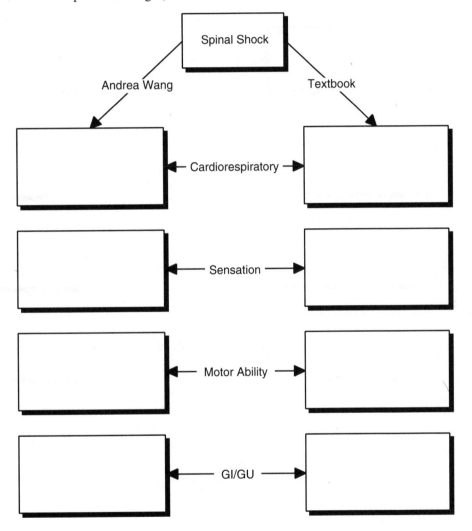

➡ Review the nurses' notes in Andrea Wang's chart for Thursday at 2000.

7. Complete the chart below to illustrate how Andrea Wang's assessment data from the Thursday 2000 nurses' notes compare with the expected findings for autonomic dysreflexia identified in your textbook.

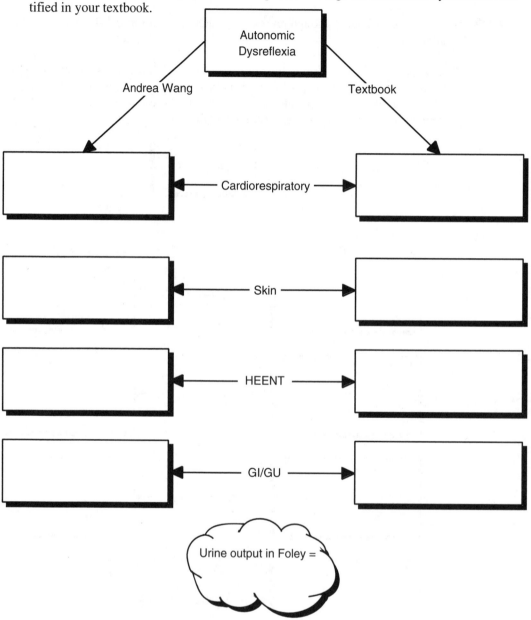

Analysis

8. Review your chart in question 7 above. Do you consider Andrea Wang's heart rate and blood pressure to be evidence of spinal shock? Explain.

9. What further data might make you more confident in your answer to question 8?

10. Identify the two priority collaborative problems or nursing diagnoses for a patient with spinal shock.

11. What is the priority nursing diagnosis for a patient with autonomic dysreflexia?

Planning/Implementation

12. In the left column below, list the nursing diagnoses and collaborative problems you identified in questions 10 and 11. (Leave plenty of space between entries.) For each entry, select one or two expected outcomes for Andrea Wang. (Refer to your textbook or an NOC manual for outcomes.) Next, offer appropriate nursing interventions for the outcomes. (Consult your textbook or an NIC manual for interventions.) Finally, provide rationales to explain how these interventions will help to achieve the expected outcomes.

Nursing Diagnosis/ Collaborative Problem	Expected Outcome(s)	Nursing Interventions	Rationale

Evaluation

 Review Andrea Wang's EPR for vital signs and assessment data. Also review her chart as needed to answer question 13.

13. In the left-hand column below, record Andrea Wang's vital signs and physical assessment findings at the time of her admission. Begin by looking in the Emergency Department Record in her Physical & History (Sunday 1230). For data not included there, scroll down to the History and Physical section (Sunday 1600). Check all pages to find the data you need. In the right-hand column, record the data found in the EPR for Thursday 1600. (Use **NM** for any data not recorded.)

	Chart Data Sunday 1230/1600	**EPR Data Thursday 1600**
Temperature		
Heart rate		
Blood pressure		
Respiratory rate		
Pain rating, source, characteristics		
Capillary refill		
Respiratory pattern		
Lung sounds		
Sensation/motion		
Bowel sounds		
GU		

14. Based on your comparisons in question 13, how successful have interventions to ensure adequate tissue oxygenation for Andrea Wang been to this point? What specific data support your analysis?

→ Return to Andrea Wang's EPR. This time check her vital signs and assessment data recorded on Thursday at 2000. Also review the nurses' notes in her chart for the same day and time.

15. For each vital sign or physical assessment area listed below, record your findings from the EPR and chart on Thursday at 2000. (Use **NM** for any data not recorded.)

EPR and Chart Data
Thursday 2000

Temperature

Heart rate

Blood pressure

Respiratory rate

Pain rating, source

Capillary refill

Respiratory pattern

Lung sounds

GU

→ Now locate Andrea Wang's intake and output data in the EPR (click on **I&O**).

16. Below, record and compare Andrea Wang's intake and urinary output on Thursday at 0800, 1600, 2000, and 2400. (Use **NM** for any data not recorded.)

	0800	1600	2000	2400
Intake				
Urinary output				

→ Return to Andrea Wang's chart and review the nurses' notes on Thursday at 2000.

17. Do you agree with the analysis offered in the nurses' note that Andrea Wang likely experienced an episode of autonomic dysreflexia? Support your answer from the data gathered in questions 13, 15, and 16.

Cultural Aspects of Care

👓 **Reading Assignment:** Cultural Aspects of Care (Chapter 6)
Patient: Andrea Wang, Room 310

This lesson focuses on the cultural aspects of health and how they affect the care you provide for your patient, Andrea Wang.

💿 In the Supervisor's Office, sign in to work with Andrea Wang on Tuesday at 1100. Access her EPR and review the Admissions Profile. Go to her room and observe the health history interview, focusing especially on the categories of Culture, Value/Belief, and Nutrition-Metabolic.

1. How does Andrea Wang identify herself?

2. To what ethnic slur did Andrea Wang refer in her description of herself? From whom would she be most likely to hear this slur, and why might someone make the comment?

3. Using Leininger's factors for assessing cultural persons (Table 6-1 in the textbook), identify some conflicts shared by many Asian Americans in the areas of kinship and social factors and philosophy and religious factors. You may need to refer to a sociology textbook in addition to your nursing textbook.

4. How does Andrea Wang seem to match the cultural assessment of Asian Americans?

5. What further areas should be explored with Andrea Wang for a more complete cultural assessment?

6. Andrea Wang is now a member of one of the subcultures of disability since she will have continuing difficulties with her mobility. List some ways that the acute care health environment serves to add to the difficulties of patients with impaired mobility.

7. Andrea Wang was asked whether she has any preferred foods or fluid. She mentioned several food preferences. What are they?

8. How well do the foods mentioned by Andrea Wang fit the nutritional requirements of the patient with spinal cord injury?

9. When Andrea Wang was asked about her food preferences, she referred to her culture. Why might she be thinking more about Chinese food at this time?

10. Use your favorite Internet search engine (or try *http://www.yahoo.com*) and do an Internet search using the keywords "Chinese-American food" and another search using "Asian-American food" as keywords. Be sure to use the quotation marks. Do you get a different set of sites each time, or do you get the same sites despite using different terms?

11. List some foods that are strongly identified with Asian-American culture. (Even if you are able to answer this on your own, verify your answer by going to one or more of the websites found in your Internet search in question 10. Remember that the weblinks for your textbook will also provide websites on this topic.)

12. Are Andrea Wang's food preferences consistent with what you have learned about Chinese-American culture? Explain.

13. Where did you get your information about Chinese-American foods?

14. How accurate and comprehensive do you think your information source(s) is (are)? On what do you base your opinion?

15. Identify resources within your community that could help Andrea Wang with her spinal cord injury and that, ideally, would also be familiar with her culture and food preferences.

16. If your community does not have readily accessible assistance for Andrea Wang, where can you direct the Wang family for information?

Case Management

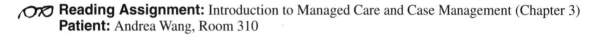 **Reading Assignment:** Introduction to Managed Care and Case Management (Chapter 3)
Patient: Andrea Wang, Room 310

In this lesson you will consider issues of case management as they apply to your patient, Andrea Wang.

 Review Chapter 3 in your textbook.

1. At what point during Andrea Wang's hospitalization would the nurse case manager become involved with her?

2. On what do you think the nurse case manager would focus during Andrea Wang's hospitalization?

3. What duties of a case manager would benefit Andrea Wang at this time?

215

4. List some likely health care team members with whom the case manager will need to coordinate care.

5. Would the case manager working with Andrea Wang more likely be an internal case manager or an external case manager? Explain.

6. Does Andrea Wang qualify for assignment to an external case manager who is working with disease state management? If so, what credentials might the nurse case manager have? Use Table 3-2 in your textbook for further information.

7. What elements should be included for an interdisciplinary clinical pathway for Andrea Wang until she is transferred to the rehabilitation unit? Your textbook contains several examples of clinical pathways. You will also find information about clinical pathways on the Simon site. (*http://www.wbsaunders.com/SIMON/Iggy/*).

8. Who is responsible for developing the clinical pathway for a given condition?

9. Discuss what will happen if Andrea Wang does not achieve the expected outcomes specified on the clinical pathway.

10. Explain continuous quality improvement as it relates to health care.

LESSON 33

Rehabilitation

👓 **Reading Assignment:** Rehabilitation Concepts for Acute and Chronic Problems
(Chapter 10)
Patient: Andrea Wang, Room 310

Your patient, Andrea Wang, is ready to be transferred from the medical-surgical floor to the rehabilitation unit. As her nurse, you need to understand the concepts of rehabilitation and how they apply directly to your patient.

💿 Please go to the Supervisor's Office and sign in to care for Andrea Wang on Thursday at 1100. Access and review her chart, EPR, and other data as needed to complete the questions in this lesson.

1. What are the overall goals of rehabilitation for chronic illness or disability?

📖 2. According to your textbook, what is rehabilitation?

3. Explain the difference between the terms *impairment*, *disability*, and *handicap*.

4. What advantages do group homes offer patients with disabilities?

5. Do you anticipate that Andrea Wang might require a group home setting in the future? Explain.

6. Given the usual membership of the rehabilitation team, which team members do you believe Andrea Wang will need the most?

 7. Using Chart 10-1 in your textbook, entitled Focused Assessment: Physical Assessment of Clients Undergoing Rehabilitation, which assessment areas are especially critical for Andrea Wang, given her SCI?

8. Summarize how you think Andrea Wang would score on the Katz Index of Activities of Daily Living as she enters the rehabilitation unit.

9. How do you think Andrea Wang should score at the point of discharge from the rehabilitation unit?

10. Review the plan of care you developed for Andrea Wang in Lesson 29, question 24. Has the focus of the plan of care for impaired mobility and altered elimination changed from that used in the acute care setting? Explain.

11. For each nursing diagnosis listed below, illustrate specifically how the plan of care for Andrea Wang has changed. List the expected outcomes and interventions you identified for acute care and those appropriate for rehabilitation.

Nursing Diagnosis	Acute Care		Rehabilitation	
	Expected Outcomes	Interventions	Expected Outcomes	Interventions
Impaired physical mobility				
Altered urination				

12. Among other issues, patients newly experiencing a chronic disability may have difficulty coping with the changes in their lives. What evidence does Andrea Wang relate during her health interview that supports the diagnosis of Ineffective individual coping?

13. Andrea Wang states that she is not sure what will happen to her relationship with her boyfriend Eric. The social worker mentions in her report that she is concerned about sexual functioning and wonders what impact her injury will have on the intimate area of her relationship with Eric. What strategies can the rehabilitation nurse implement to assist the patient in this matter?

14. What strategies should be implemented prior to the patient's discharge from the rehabilitation unit to facilitate the transfer from institutional living to community and independent living?

Community-Based Care

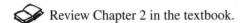 **Reading Assignment:** Community-Based Care (Chapter 2)
Patient: Andrea Wang, Room 310

In this lesson, you will consider the community-based care needs of your patient, Andrea Wang.

Review Chapter 2 in the textbook.

1. What type of care is Andrea Wang planning to use after discharge?

2. What major responsibility of the nurse in ambulatory care will Andrea Wang need?

Sign in to work with Andrea Wang for the Thursday 1100 shift. Attend the health team meeting in Conference Room 2 (Room 308) and listen to each team member's report.

3. What are the principal concerns of the nurse case manager regarding discharge planning for Andrea Wang?

4. What is the clinical nurse specialist's major concern about Andrea Wang's discharge plan?

225

5. Identify the main concerns that the social worker has about Andrea Wang's discharge plan.

6. Are the needs and concerns identified by the health team members appropriate for management by a nurse in ambulatory care at this time? Explain.

 Review the community-based care and teaching needed by the patient with a spinal cord injury. (See Chapter 43 in your textbook.)

7. Using the textbook and your answers to questions 3, 4, and 5, complete the chart below.

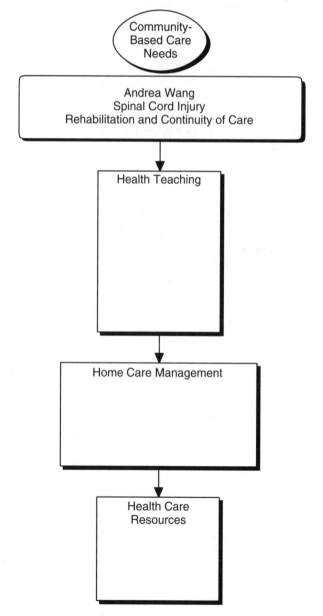

8. What information should be included in a discharge plan for Andrea Wang to attempt to prevent future infections?

9. Families of patients newly experiencing a chronic disability may have difficulty coping with the changes in their family member's life, as well as in their own lives. What evidence might the home care nurse find to indicate that Andrea Wang's family is experiencing difficulties in coping?

10. Some families rise more quickly to the challenges of coping with health crises. What evidence might the home care nurse find that would indicate that Andrea Wang's family members are coping with the challenges and are ready for further growth?

11. Based on the items you identified for inclusion in a plan of care for Andrea Wang in the community, what are some outcome measures that you would want to document?

Evaluation of Care

Reading Assignment: Interventions for Clients with Problems of the Central Nervous System: The Spinal Cord (Chapter 43)

Patient: Andrea Wang, Room 310

Andrea Wang will soon be discharged to the rehabilitation unit. As her nurse, it will be your responsibility to make sure that she has all the needed information regarding her immediate care after transfer.

Please go to the Supervisor's Office and sign in to care for Andrea Wang on Thursday at 1100. Attend the health team meeting in Conference Room 2 (Room 308).

1. What are the overall goals for the care of patients with a spinal cord injury?

2. What information needs to be included in a transfer nurse's note for Andrea Wang's medical record, assuming that the rehabilitation unit is located away from the medical center?

3. The nurse case manager and the social worker both express concern about Andrea Wang's coping ability, as well as her family's ability to cope with her condition. Identify at least two factors that almost certainly will affect the course of her rehabilitation.

4. What information about the rehabilitation unit should be given to Andrea Wang?

 5. In Chapter 43 of your textbook, review the evaluation outcomes for spinal cord injury. In the left column below, list the expected outcomes suggested. (You will complete the other columns in question 6.)

Expected Outcomes	Nurses' Notes	Physicians' Notes	EPR
Spinal cord injury			

Go to the Nurses' Station and open Andrea Wang's chart. Review the nurses' notes and physicians' notes, looking for evidence that indicates whether or not the outcomes suggested by your textbook have been achieved in her case. Then access her EPR and search for the same evidence in her data summaries.

6. Record your findings on the chart in question 5 on the previous page. Next to each outcome, under the corresponding CD source of data, record a **Y** if you found evidence of outcome attainment, record an **N** if you found evidence that the outcome had not been achieved, and record **NM** if the outcome was not mentioned.

7. Based on your chart in question 5, what outcomes need to be evaluated and noted?

8. Now that you have reviewed Andrea Wang's data and considered the health team members' concerns for her, are there any problems or events that should be added to the evaluation of her care during this time? If so, explain.

9. How might the nurse discharging Andrea Wang ensure continuing evaluation of any problems identified in question 8?

LESSON **36** _____

Infection

_____

 Reading Assignment: Interventions for Clients with Infection (Chapter 26)
Patients: Carmen Gonzales, Room 302
David Ruskin, Room 303

In this lesson, you will focus on infection and its effect on two patients, Carmen Gonzales and David Ruskin. To refamiliarize yourself with these cases, review previous lessons in Parts I and IV, especially Lessons 2 and 22.

Before you begin working with the patients, read Chapter 26 in your textbook.

Pathophysiology

1. What elements are necessary for an infection to occur?

2. Explain the difference between virulence and pathogenicity.

Access Carmen Gonzales' and David Ruskin's data on your CD-ROM as needed to answer the following questions. Remember that you can work with only one patient at a time. To switch patients, you will need to return to the Supervisor's Office, click on the desktop computer, click **Reset**, and select the new patient. Use Tuesday 0700 as your sign-in time for both patients. You will need to review the Physical & History in each patient's chart (Remember to scroll down to read all pages.) Also review each patient's Admissions Profile, laboratory results, and other data summaries in the EPR.

3. Based on your review of the patients' data, complete the illustrations below, comparing the events in the chain of infection for Carmen Gonzales and David Ruskin. Refer to Figure 26-1 in your textbook for guidance. If any information requested in the diagrams is not clearly indicated in the patient's data, record your best estimate.

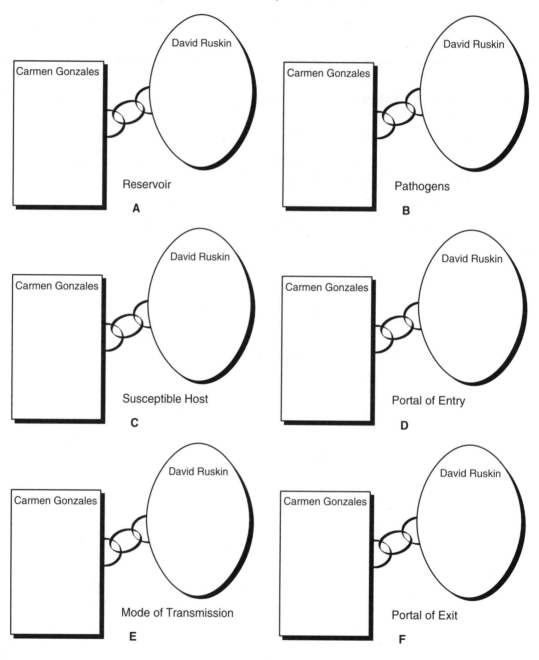

4. Considering the clinical information available to you, which of your two patients is the most susceptible to infection at this time? Why?

5. How may age be a factor for Carmen Gonzales?

6. What evidence does each patient exhibit that indicates the body is using *nonspecific* defenses against infection?

7. What evidence does each patient exhibit that indicates the body is using *specific* defenses against infection?

8. What is the single most effective method of infection control, both in the hospital and in the community?

9. Do either Carmen Gonzales or David Ruskin need additional precautions beyond the Center for Disease Control's Universal Precautions? Why or why not?

10. What data should cause the infection control nurse to order contact precautions for Carmen Gonzales?

11. As you plan your activities, you realize that both Carmen Gonzales and David Ruskin need a dressing change. Should one patient's dressing be changed before the other? If so, whose? Explain your answer.

12. If gender were not an issue (that is, if Carmen Gonzales and David Ruskin were of the same sex), would there be any reason they should not share a room? Explain.

13. You are assisting David Ruskin's orthopedic surgeon, Dr. Frank Renfro, with a dressing change. The surgeon walks into the room, greets the patient, pulls down his hospital gown, and removes the surgical dressing. He then observes the wound, pokes lightly at the flesh around the staples, and leaves the room after telling you to apply a dry sterile dressing. You noted that Dr. Renfro did not wash his hands before removing the dressing, did not use sterile gloves to palpate the area around the sutures, and did not wash his hands before he left the room. What should you do? Explain.

14. How might you handle a similar situation in the future?

15. You step out of David Ruskin's room in time to see Sharon Saunders, a patient care assistant (PCA) leaving Carmen Gonzales' room and walking toward the clean linen cart while wearing disposable gloves. What should you do?

16. A short time later, you observe the PCA making David Ruskin's bed. She drops the soiled linen on the floor and places used towels and wet wash clothes on the chair next to the patient's bed. What should you do? Why?

17. Later in your shift, you observe the PCA again leaving Carmen Gonzales' room and walking down the corridor with gloves on, this time carrying soiled linen in her arms next to her body. What should you do? Why?

Assessment

18. Complete the chart below to compare the key features of infection for David Ruskin and Carmen Gonzales. Using your textbook as a guide, list the common symptoms of infection in the center column of boxes. To the right of each box, record David Ruskin's symptoms. List Carmen Gonzales' symptoms on the left.

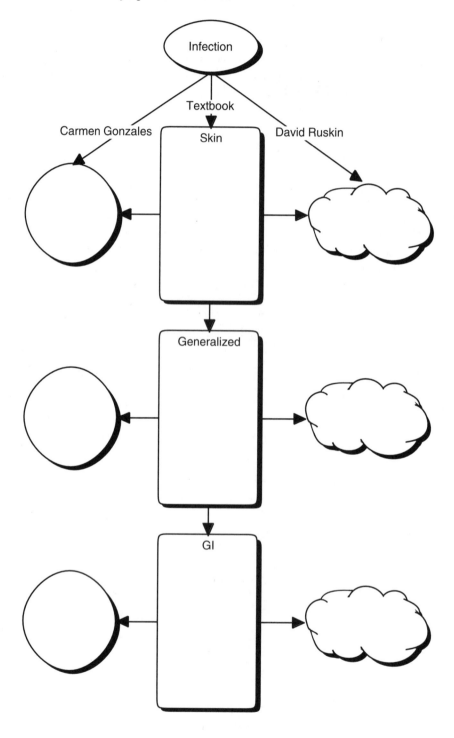

→ Review data provided on your CD-ROM as needed to answer question 19. (Hint: Try the diagnostics section of the patients' charts and the data summaries in the EPR.

19. Complete the chart below to indicate which diagnostic tests were performed for Carmen Gonzales and David Ruskin to determine the presence of microorganisms. For each test listed in the center column of boxes, identify the normal values. (You may need to consult a laboratory diagnostics manual for these values.) To the left and right of each test, indicate whether or not that test was performed for each patient. Include results for any tests that were performed.

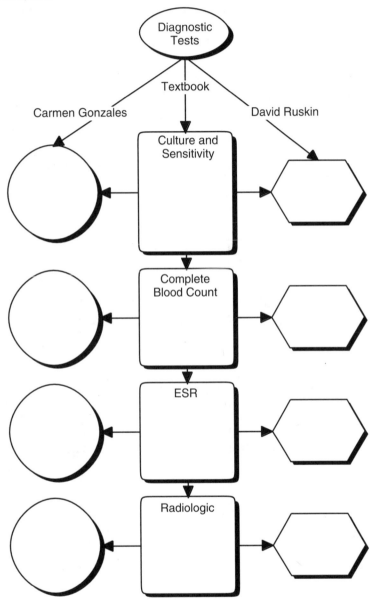

Analysis

20. Based on your findings concerning infection, what nursing diagnoses or collaborative problems would you select for Carmen Gonzales?

21. What nursing diagnoses or collaborative problems would you select for David Ruskin?

Review the physicians' orders in both patients' charts.

Planning/Implementation

22. Complete the chart below to identify the interventions for infection that were ordered for Carmen Gonzales and David Ruskin. In the center column, for each complication listed, identify interventions suggested by your textbook. To the left and right, indicate what specific interventions were ordered for each patient.

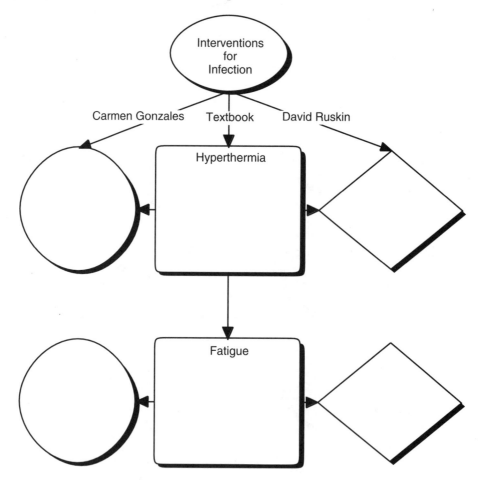

Evaluation

 23. Review the expected outcomes for infection in Chapter 26 of your textbook. In the left column below, list the expected outcomes suggested. (You will fill in the other columns in question 24.)

Expected Outcomes	Nurses' Notes	Physicians' Notes	EPR
Infection			

➤ In Carmen Gonzales' and David Ruskin's charts, review the nurses' notes and physicians' notes, looking for evidence that indicates whether or not the outcomes for infection suggested by your textbook have been achieved in either or both of their cases. Then access the EPR and search for the same evidence in their data summaries.

24. Record your findings on the chart in question 23 above. Next to each outcome, under the corresponding CD source of data, record a **Y** if you found evidence of outcome attainment, record an **N** if you found evidence that the outcome had not been achieved, and record **NM** if the outcome was not mentioned. For answers that apply to only one of the patients, indicate by including the patient's initials—CG or DR.

25. What major area of infection control needs to be implemented for both patients?

26. Considering the observations you have made in this lesson, what suggestions can you make that will improve infection control measures on your unit? What follow-up activities can you suggest that will help keep infection control awareness high?

Continuing Care

27. What general household measures to control infection do Carmen Gonzales' family and David Ruskin's family need to consider?

28. Carmen Gonzales may be on antibiotic therapy for a time after she is discharged home. What measures should the home care nurse plan to teach the patient and her family?

LESSON **37** ────────────────────

Oxygenation

──

 Reading Assignment: Assessment of the Respiratory System (Chapter 27)
Interventions for Critically Ill Patients with Respiratory Problems
(Chapter 32)
Patients: Sally Begay, Room 302
Ira Bradley, Room 309

For this lesson, you will consider issues of oxygenation and how they affect the health of Sally
Begay and Ira Bradley.

Before you begin working with your patients, read Chapter 32 in your textbook. Also review
Chapter 27 as needed.

Assessment

1. What history data should the nurse record for any patient experiencing difficulties with oxygenation?

2. What are the respiratory changes associated with aging?

3. Are the age-related respiratory changes considered "normal"? Explain.

To complete question 4, you will need to review the Physical & History for Sally Begay and Ira Bradley in the patient charts. For each patient, sign in for the Tuesday 1100 shift.

4. In the chart below, compare Sally Begay's and Ira Bradley's history assessment data in relation to oxygenation. Using your textbook as a guide, record the normal findings for each history area listed in the center column. In the side boxes, record the findings you located for each patient.

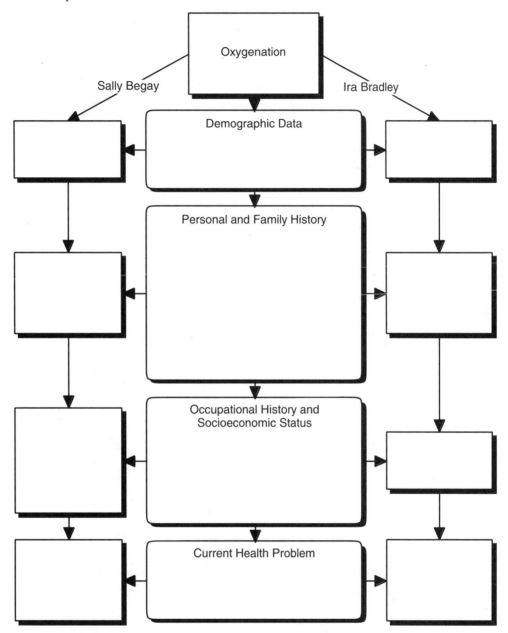

→ Access each patient's EPR and review all data related to oxygenation and/or respiratory assessment.

5. In the chart below, compare Sally Begay's and Ira Bradley's respiratory physical assessment data. Consult your textbook and record normal findings for each area listed in the center boxes. In the side boxes, record specific findings for each patient.

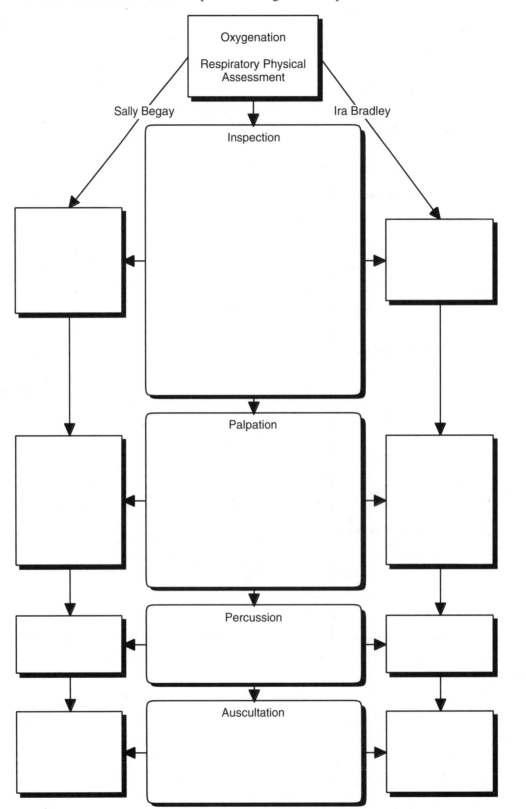

➤ Review each patient's EPR and chart data, including diagnostic reports, as needed to answer question 6.

6. In the chart below, compare Sally Begay's and Ira Bradley's respiratory diagnostic assessment data. Using your textbook as a guide, identify the diagnostic tests normally orderd for each category listed in the center boxes. In the side boxes, indicate whether these tests were done for each patient. Include results for any tests that were performed.

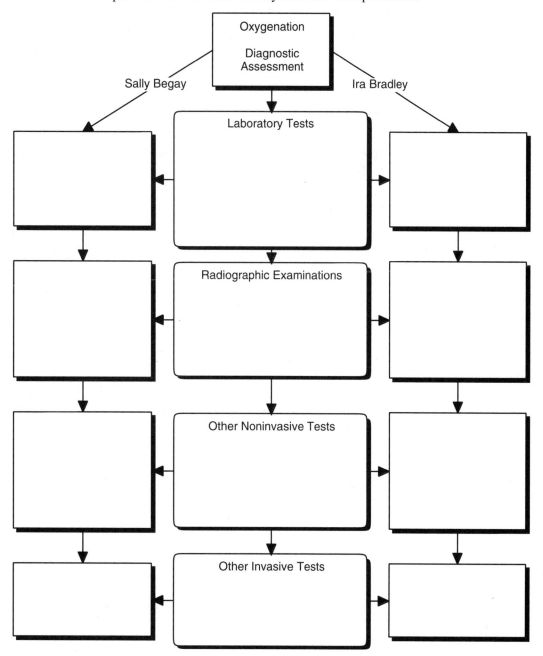

7. Review your answers to question 4. Formulate questions for data that are missing from Sally Begay's history.

8. Formulate questions for data that are missing from Ira Bradley's history.

9. Based on your answers to question 5, what further physical assessments of Sally Begay should be done to complete her respiratory physical assessment?

10. What further physical assessments of Ira Bradley should be done to complete his respiratory physical assessment?

11. Review your answers to question 6. What further diagnostic tests, if any, do you think should be ordered for Sally Begay? For Ira Bradley?

Analysis

→ 12. Using your textbook as a guide, fill in the center column of the chart below, identifying the clinical indicators of hypoxia for each area listed. In the side boxes, record your assessment findings for Sally Begay and Ira Bradley. (Review data available on your CD-ROM as needed.)

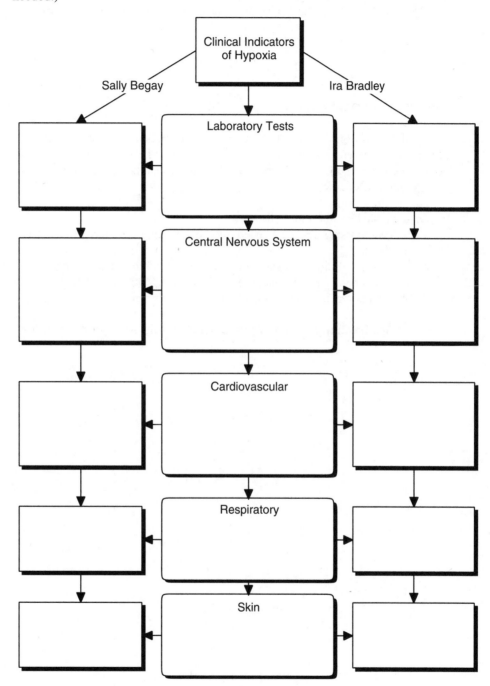

13. State the difference between hypoxemia and hypoxia.

14. Do either Sally Begay or Ira Bradley meet the criteria for hypoxemia? Explain your answer.

15. Do either Sally Begay or Ira Bradley meet the criteria for hypoxia? Give your rationale.

Planning/Implementation

To complete questions 16 annd 17, you will need to consult a nursing diagnosis handbook—ideally one that adheres to NANDA nomenclature. You will also need three different colored highlighters. (You may substitute colors other than those specified in the instructions—as long as you use three different colors.)

16. On the table below, do the following:
 a. For each nursing diagnosis listed, record defining characteristics as identified in your handbook.
 b. Circle any defining characteristics that appear in more than one column.
 c. Mark all characteristics that apply to Sally Begay with a pink highlighter.
 d. Mark all characteristics that apply to Ira Bradley with a blue highlighter.

Impaired Gas Exchange	Ineffective Breathing Pattern	Ineffective Airway Clearance

17. Based on your chart in question 16, which nursing diagnoses are appropriate for Sally Begay? For Ira Bradley? Explain your answers.

18. Identify at least ten interventions that nurses commonly use for patients with respiratory problems. Do not limit yourself to interventions appropriate for the patients in this lesson. Use your textbook and an NIC manual for ideas.

19. Which interventions would you choose for Sally Begay?

20. Which interventions would you choose for Ira Bradley?

21. What pharmacologic measures may be used to improve oxygenation?

22. Given her medical diagnoses, what pharmacologic therapy can you expect to be ordered for Sally Begay?

23. Given Ira Bradley's medical diagnoses, what pharmacologic therapy can you expect?

Community Care

24. Identify four teaching items that all patients with lower respiratory disease need for illness prevention.

Ira Bradley & David Ruskin

LESSON **38** _____

Central Nervous System

_____

 Reading Assignment: Interventions for Critically Ill Clients with Neurologic Problems
(Chapter 45)
Patients: Ira Bradley, Room 309
David Ruskin, Room 303

For this lesson, you will focus on issues related to the central nervous system as they apply to
Ira Bradley and David Ruskin. You may find it helpful to refer to your answers in previous
lessons, especially Lessons 15 and 23.

Access and review Ira Bradley's and David Ruskin's data as needed to complete the exercises in
this lesson. Use Thursday 1100 as your shift for the entire lesson.

Review Chapter 45 in your textbook.

Physiology

1. Ira Bradley and David Ruskin both have a history of head injury. Describe the sequence of
    events leading from head injury to increased intracranial pressure.

2. Using the Monroe-Kellie doctrine, explain why increased intracranial pressure is of concern.

3. Explain how increased intracranial pressure causes damage to brain cells.

4. Complete the chart below to compare the clinical manifestations of late increased intracranial pressure and the clinical manifestations expected for the progressive stage of shock. (Consult your textbook if you need help.)

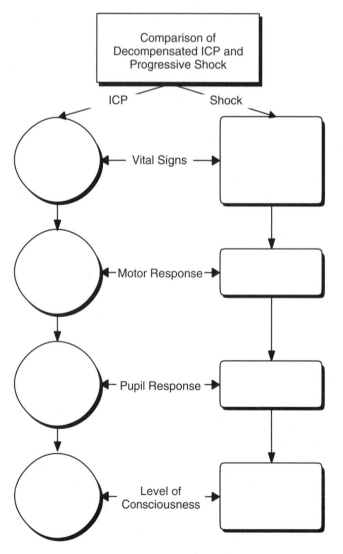

5. What risk factors does Ira Bradley have for ICP?

6. What risk factors does David Ruskin have for ICP?

Assessment

7. What evidence does each patient exhibit on admission that indicates he may be experiencing ICP? Use the graphic below to record your answers.

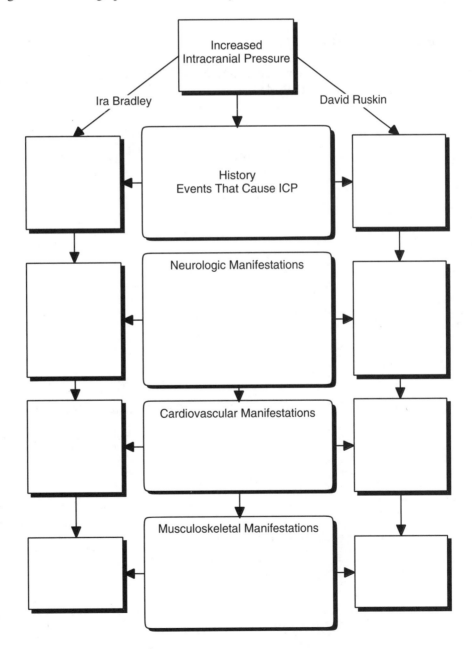

Analysis

8. Do you think that either Ira Bradley or David Ruskin shows evidence of ICP? If so, who? Explain your answer.

9. At what stage of ICP, if any, would either patient probably be placed? Explain your answer.

Planning/Implementation

10. What is one of the most important responsibilities of the nurse in caring for patients such as Ira Bradley and David Ruskin?

11. What nursing or patient activities may increase ICP?

12. What effect does hypoventilation have on ICP?

13. What is the major therapeutic goal once ICP has been identified?

14. Identify the collaborative interventions for ICP.

15. Briefly state the purpose for each of the drug classes used to manage ICP. Use the table below to record your answer.

Drug Class	Purposee
Barbiturates (phentobarbital sodium)	
Osmotic diuretics	
Loop diuretics	
Narcotics (codeine or fentanyl)	
Neuromuscular blocking agents	
Anticonvulsants	

16. Identify one nursing diagnosis and one collaborative problem appropriate for ICP.

17. In the left column below, list the nursing diagnosis and collaborative problem you identified in question 16. For each entry, write two expected outcomes and several nursing interventions. Provide rationales for your interventions. Use your textbok and refer to NOC and NIC manuals for additional suggestions.

Nursing Diagnosis/ Collaborative Problem	Expected Outcomes	Nursing Interventions	Rationale

Evaluation

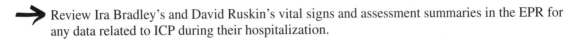 Review Ira Bradley's and David Ruskin's vital signs and assessment summaries in the EPR for any data related to ICP during their hospitalization.

18. Based on your review of the EPR data, how successful have nursing measures been to prevent ICP in Ira Bradley and David Ruskin? What evidence do you have to support your evaluation?

Community-Based Care

19. What information will Ira Bradley's wife need to monitor her husband's functioning at home?

20. What information will Mrs. Ruskin need to monitor her husband's functioning when he returns home?

LESSON **39** _____

Adult Development

_____

ᴏᴏ **Reading Assignment:** Health Care of Older Adults (Chapter 5)
Patients: Sally Begay, Room 304
   Andrea Wang, Room 310

In this lesson, you will focus on issues of adult development as they apply to Sally Begay and Andrea Wang. To refamiliarize yourself with these patients' cases, review your answers to previous lessons in Parts II and V, especially Lessons 8 and 29.

Review Sally Begay's and Andrea Wang's data as needed to answer the questions in this lesson. Use Tuesday 1100 as your shift when you sign in to care for either patient. Remember, you can only access data and care for one patient at a time.

Briefly review Chapter 5 in your textbook. You may also need to review concepts of adult development in a fundamentals of nursing textbook or a growth and development textbook.

Assessment

1. Identify six elements that are usually assessed to determine an individual's development.

2. What other assessments of developmental status are especially pertinent to nurses during the care planning process?

Analysis

3. Compare Andrea Wang's and Sally Begay's stages of development on the chart below.

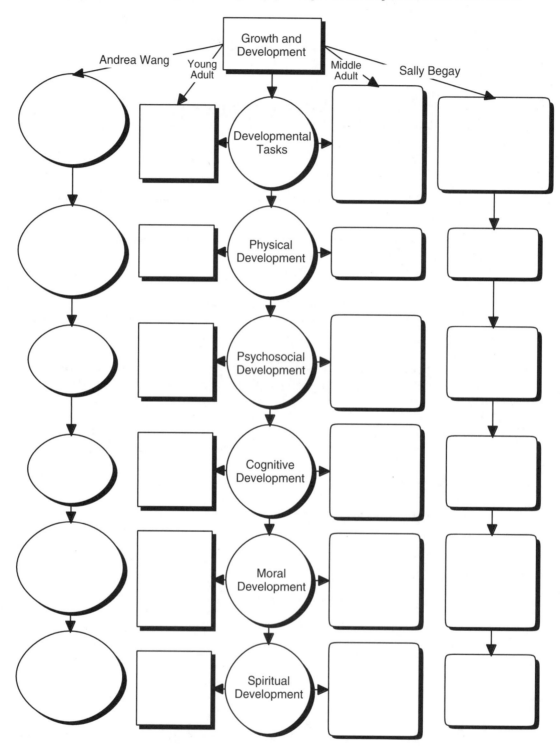

4. Complete the chart below to show how Andrea Wang and Sally Begay compare with the normal growth and development patterns for their stage with regard to health problems.

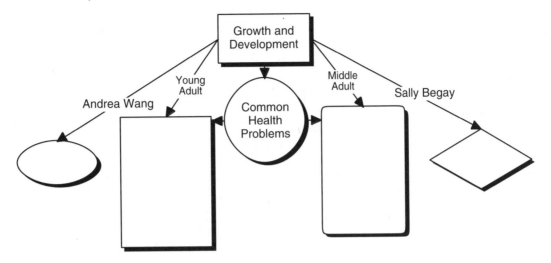

5. What is the leading cause of death in young adults?

6. What is the leading cause of death in the middle adult age group?

7. What are the common health problems of older adults?

8. Considering the common health problems of young adults, for what health problems is Andrea Wang particularly at risk? Provide rationales for your choices.

9. Considering the common health problems of middle adults, for what health problems is Sally Begay particularly at risk? Provide rationales.

10. What health promotion activities are appropriate for Andrea Wang with regard to the normal growth and development patterns for her stage? Which are appropriate for Sally Begay? Use the chart below to record your answers.

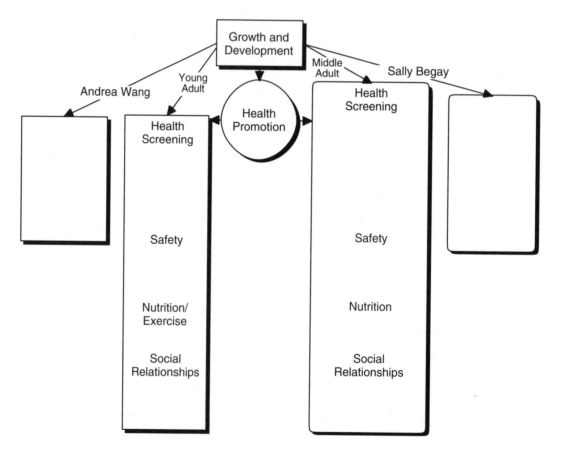

11. Of the health promotion activities you identified as appropriate for Andrea Wang and Sally Begay, in which do each of them engage? Record your answers on the chart in question 10.

12. What are five health-protecting activities that are appropriate for older adults?

13. What are five health-enhancing behaviors that are appropriate for older adults?

14. Based on what you have learned about Andrea Wang and Sally Begay, were they meeting their expected developmental tasks at the time of their hospitalization? Provide supporting evidence for your answers.

Planning/Implementation

15. Which patient is most at risk for delayed growth and development? Explain.

16. What nursing diagnoses should be included for Andrea Wang? Base your answer on her current health problems, your analysis of her stage of development status, and the common health problems for her stage.

17. What nursing diagnoses should be included for Sally Begay? Base you answer upon her current health problems, your analysis of her stage of development status, and the common health problems for her stage.

18. Develop a plan of care for Andrea Wang for the nursing diagnosis Risk for delayed growth and development. In the table below, identify your expected outcomes for this diagnosis, appropriate interventions to achieve those outcomes, and rationales for your interventions. Use your textbook or and refer to NIC and NOC manuals for additional help.

Plan of Care: Risk for Delayed Growth and Development

Expected Outcomes	Nursing Interventions	Rationales

19. Develop a plan of care for Sally Begay for the nursing diagnosis Ineffective health mainte-nance. Provide expected outcomes, interventions, and rationales below.

Plan of Care: Ineffective Health Maintenance

Expected Outcomes	Nursing Interventions	Rationales

Evaluation

20. At what point(s) would you plan to evaluate the success of your plan of care for Risk for delayed growth and development for Andrea Wang?

21. At what point(s) would you plan to evaluate the success of your plan of care for Ineffective health maintenance for Sally Begay?

Community-Based Care

22. What is the responsibility of the home care nurse for evaluating Andrea Wang's progress in young adult development?

23. What is the responsibility of the home care nurse for evaluation Sally Begay's health maintenance activities?

LESSON 40 ————————————————————

Shock

————————————————————

/∞ **Reading Assignment:** Interventions for Clients With Shock (Chapter 37)
Patients: Carmen Gonzales, Room 302
Andrea Wang, Room 310

In this lesson, you will focus on shock and its potential effect on the health of Carmen Gonzales and Andrea Wang. You may find it helpful to review your answers to previous lessons in Parts II and V, especially Lessons 2 and 29.

Access and review data on the CD-ROM as needed to complete the exercises in this lesson. Remember, you can only work with one patient at a time. Select the Thursday 1100 shift when you sign in for either patient.

Review Chapter 37 in your textbook.

Physiology

1. Describe the underlying abnormal cellular metabolism that is central to all forms of shock.

2. Using the new classification system described in your textbook, describe the functional impairment causing neurally induced distributive shock.

3. Using the new classification system, describe the functional impairment causing chemically induced distributive shock.

4. Complete the chart below to show the physiology of the four stages of shock and the clinical manifestations expected for each stage of shock. Consult your textbook for suggestions.

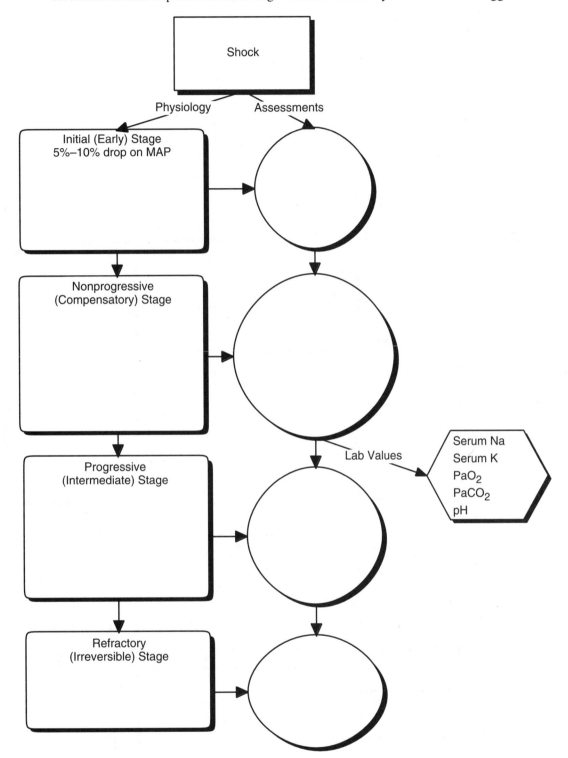

5. What risk factors does Carmen Gonzales have for shock? What type of shock is she most likely to experience?

6. What risk factors does Andrea Wang have for shock? What type of shock is she most likely to experience?

Assessment

7. What evidence does each patient exhibit on admission that indicates she may be experiencing shock? Record your answers on the chart below.

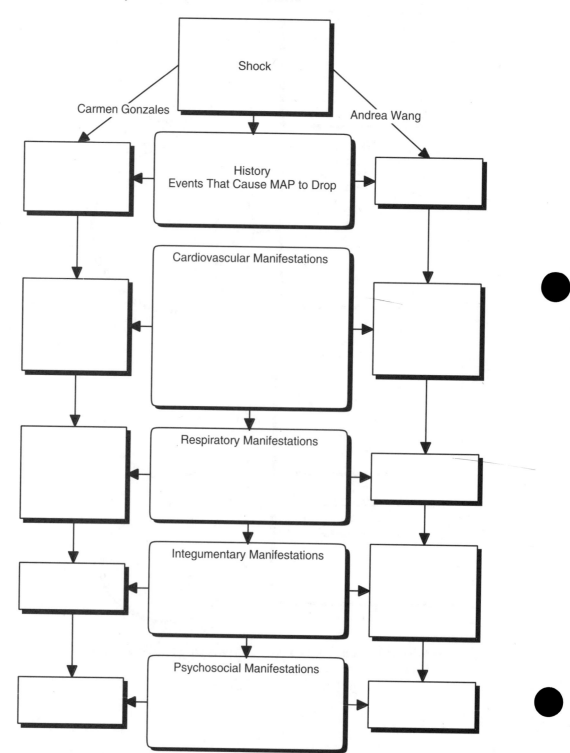

Analysis

8. Do you think that either patient shows evidence of shock? If so, who? Explain your answer.

9. At what stage of shock, if any, would either Andrea Wang or Carmen Gonzales probably be placed? Explain your answer.

Planning/Implementation

10. What is one of the most important responsibilities of the nurse in caring for patients such as Carmen Gonzales and Andrea Wang?

11. What is the major therapeutic intervention once shock has been identified?

12. What are the collaborative interventions for chemically induced distributive or septic shock?

13. What are the collaborative interventions for neurally induced distributive or spinal shock?

14. What nursing diagnoses or collaborative problems are appropriate for distributive shock?

 15. Develop a plan of care for the collaborative problem Potential for MODS. In the table below, identify two expected outcomes for the problem, nursing interventions to achieve those outcomes, and rationales for your interventions. Consult your textbook for help. Refer to NIC and NOC manuals for additional interventions and outcomes.

Plan of Care: CP: Potential for MODS

Expected Outcomes	Nursing Interventions	Rationales

For both Carmen Gonzales and Andrea Wang, check the EPR data (from admission to the present) for any findings related to distributive shock.

Evaluation

16. Based on your review of the EPR data, how successful have nursing measures been to prevent distributive shock in these patients? What evidence do you have to support your evaluation?

Community-Based Care

17. What information will Carmen Gonzales need to remain free of sepsis when she returns home?

18. What information will Andrea Wang need to remain free of sepsis when she returns home?

19. What specific assessments should the home health nurse make during visits to Carmen Gonzales? (Hint: Refer to Chart 37-10 in your textbook.)